Healthcare Quality Measurement

Volume 2: Statistical Methodology

This comprehensive guide presents a data science approach to healthcare quality measurement and provider profiling for policymakers, regulators, hospital quality leaders, clinicians, and researchers. Two volumes encompass basic and advanced statistical techniques and diverse practical applications.

Volume 1 begins with a historical review followed by core concepts including measure types and attributes (bias, validity, reliability, power, and sample size); data sources; target conditions and procedures; patient and provider observation periods; attribution level; risk modeling; social risk factors; outlier classification; data presentation; public reporting; and graphical approaches.

Volume 2 introduces causal inference for provider profiling, focusing on hierarchical regression models. These models appropriately partition systematic and random variation in observations, accounting for within-provider clustering. Item response theory models are introduced for linking multiple categorical quality metrics to underlying quality constructs. Computational strategies are discussed, followed by various approaches to inference. Finally, methods to assess and compare model fit are presented.

Sharon-Lise T. Normand is S. James Adelstein Professor of Health Care Policy at Harvard University. She is an authority on the statistical methodology for hierarchical observational data, playing an essential role in emphasizing the importance of statistics in assessing the quality of healthcare. She is Fellow of the American Statistical Association (ASA), American College of Cardiology (ACC), American Heart Association (AHA), and American Association for the Advancement of Science (AAAS).

David M. Shahian is Professor of Surgery at Harvard Medical School. With his background as a cardiac surgeon, department chair, and health services researcher, he has been a pioneering leader in healthcare quality measurement and public reporting initiatives at the state and national levels. He has served on the National Quality Forum Board and Executive Committee and was Vice President of Quality and Safety at Massachusetts General Hospital.

"This two-volume compendium from two titans in the field of healthcare quality measurement at MGH and Harvard will be a go-to reference on properly assessing healthcare quality. And a key aspect of properly assessing quality is causal inference, which is covered comprehensively in the two volumes."

Mike Daniels, ***Professor and Andrew Banks Family Endowed Chair, Department of Statistics, University of Florida***

"Assessing the quality of healthcare is an incredibly important—and incredibly challenging—topic; doing so well can help ensure high-quality care and save resources. This book provides a rigorous and comprehensive overview of this vast field, with an important focus on the inherent causal questions involved. It will be an important resource both for those new to the field as well as to those steeped in these topics, sure to be pulled off of bookshelves frequently!"

Elizabeth Stuart, ***Frank Hurley and Catharine Dorrier Professor and Chair, Department of Biostatistics, Bloomberg School of Public Health, Johns Hopkins University***

"Healthcare Quality Measurement by Normand and Shahian is the definitive, rigorous guide to measuring healthcare performance. Blending statistical depth with real-world insight, it brings order to a fragmented field and sets a new standard for validity, transparency, and responsible use of quality metrics."

Harlan Krumholz, MD, SM, ***Harold H. Hines, Jr. Professor of Medicine (Cardiology), Yale School of Medicine, and Director, Yale Center for Outcomes Research and Evaluation (CORE)***

Healthcare Quality Measurement

Volume 2: Statistical Methodology

Sharon-Lise T. Normand

Harvard Medical School

David M. Shahian

Harvard Medical School

CAMBRIDGE
UNIVERSITY PRESS

CAMBRIDGE
UNIVERSITY PRESS

Shaftesbury Road, Cambridge CB2 8EA, United Kingdom

One Liberty Plaza, 20th Floor, New York, NY 10006, USA

477 Williamstown Road, Port Melbourne, VIC 3207, Australia

314–321, 3rd Floor, Plot 3, Splendor Forum, Jasola District Centre,
New Delhi – 110025, India

Cambridge University Press is part of Cambridge University Press & Assessment,
a department of the University of Cambridge.

We share the University's mission to contribute to society through the pursuit of
education, learning and research at the highest international levels of excellence.

www.cambridge.org
Information on this title: www.cambridge.org/9781009648158
DOI: 10.1017/9781009648196

When citing this work, please include a reference to the DOI 10.1017/9781009648196

First published 2026

A catalogue record for this publication is available from the British Library

A Cataloging-in-Publication data record for this book is available from the Library of Congress

ISBN 978-1-009-64815-8 Hardback
ISBN 978-1-009-64818-9 Paperback

Contents

Contents of Volume 1

Preface and Acknowledgments

Excessive variation in provider outcomes is a pervasive challenge and opportunity for healthcare reform. Accurate measurement of healthcare quality is critical to identifying and mitigating this undesirable variation and has evolved from simple counts of deaths to comprehensive, multi-dimensional scores of processes of care and outcomes. The applications of these diverse provider quality metrics have similarly expanded. Measures such as hospital mortality, complications, adherence to recommended treatment guidelines, and patient perceptions of their care are used by health insurance companies and state and federal governments in value-based purchasing and selective contracting; by regulatory agencies to monitor and publish provider performance data; by providers to identify and remediate quality issues; and by patients to make their informed choices of providers.

Given the broad array of available quality metrics and methodologies and their diverse downstream applications, including public reporting, making appropriate healthcare quality inferences is complex, challenging, and high-stakes. Measurement of *quality* is not a simple accounting of what was done to a patient or their outcomes. Rather, observational data are used to infer the underlying quality of care of the healthcare provider based on observed outcomes, and this information must be valid and reliable. Choosing and applying appropriate statistical methodology is a critical requirement and must consider the many statistical issues associated with making inferences from observational data, such as the management of *clustering* of similar patients within providers.

The theoretical foundation for quantitatively assessing healthcare provider quality lies in *causal inference*, a fact that is often unrecognized or ignored. Measure developers commonly focus on estimating the best predictive models for patient outcomes, but their major objective should be to balance the distributions of patients' health status *across providers*, which is the goal of *risk-adjustment*. These patient risk factors must be carefully selected. For example, while some observable information will improve predictions, variables on the causal pathway should not be included. Often these decisions are obvious, but for some variables, such as a patient's race/ethnicity or other sociodemographic factors, they are not straightforward and may be controversial.

The goal of this book is to provide a comprehensive perspective on healthcare quality assessment, addressing the many statistical issues involved in making inferences about provider performance as well as the multitude of practical, regulatory, and health policy issues that arise when applying these inferences to improve healthcare quality. An important motivation for writing this book was our frustration with the generally chaotic healthcare measurement landscape in the US and internationally. Important measure design principles are often neither appreciated nor applied, and there are few if any standards to prevent the widespread use of methodologically flawed, inaccurate, and misleading metrics.

We began this project more than a decade ago. The length of time it has taken to complete reflects the complexity of the subject, its continuing evolution, and our own personal growth in knowledge and experience. We are unaware of any other book that provides a similarly comprehensive treatment of healthcare quality measurement from both the statistical and practical implementation perspectives. It should be a valuable resource (including extensive references) for readers at many levels, including premedical students; medical school and public health students and faculty; interns, residents, and fellows with an interest in quality; attending physicians and surgeons whose quality is being monitored; regulators and payers who regularly use these data; quality leaders and administrators in hospitals, other healthcare facilities, and health plans; health policy researchers; statistical faculty and students; and anyone leading healthcare quality initiatives.

To broadly encompass the topic and to provide material that will be valuable to readers at all levels, this book is separated into two parts. Volume 1 focuses on the history and evolution of healthcare quality measurement; important methodological considerations in the design, validation, and implementation of provider profiling measures; public reporting of provider performance, including both its potential value and unintended consequences; direct-to-consumer online healthcare ratings; and graphical approaches to provider profiling. Volume 2 is more technical, discussing statistical approaches in a unified, detailed fashion that will be particularly useful for those with advanced statistical training.

We have extensive experience with hospital, state, and national quality measurement and public reporting initiatives, including their positive potential and their inevitable frustrations, costs, and occasional unintended consequences. The frequent usage of cardiovascular disease exemplars in this book is no coincidence, as we have drawn upon unique domain expertise in quality measurement for cardiac surgery and percutaneous coronary interventions, both of which areas have been paradigms for the development and reporting of healthcare quality measures.

Sharon-Lise Normand has developed statistical approaches for assessing the quality of healthcare providers since 1990, focusing on Bayesian approaches to inference that facilitate the computation of estimators of complex parameters. This work was motivated by an early study of US hospital variation in mortality rates following a heart attack. Since that time, she has developed estimators of hospital quality for the Centers for Medicare and Medicaid Services and has advised the American Heart Association and the American College of Cardiology on construction of various healthcare provider measures. For more than a decade, she led the Massachusetts Data Analysis Center (Mass-DAC), a data coordinating center contracted by the Massachusetts Department of Public Health to profile all hospitals, cardiac surgeons, and coronary interventionalists performing cardiac surgery or coronary interventions. This *in the trenches* experience underscored many of the practical issues and unintended consequences with the construction of report cards.

With extensive experience as a practicing cardiac surgeon and department chair, David Shahian served for several decades as a senior leader of Society of Thoracic Surgeons (STS) cardiothoracic surgery data registries, risk model and quality measure development, public reporting initiatives, and performance improvement activities. On behalf of STS, he accepted the 2018 John M. Eisenberg Award for quality and safety from the Joint Commission and National Quality Forum. Dr. Shahian has served on or led quality-focused technical expert panels for the National Quality Forum, the Centers for Medicare and Medicaid Services, the American College of Cardiology, and the American Heart Association. As chair of the Massachusetts Cardiac Care Quality Commission, he was a leader in implementing mandatory public reporting of cardiac surgical outcomes in the Commonwealth, where he also served as president of the Massachusetts Society of Thoracic Surgeons and Vice President of the Center for Quality and Safety at the Massachusetts General Hospital. Dr. Shahian served on the Board and Executive Committee of the National Quality Forum, the inaugural Consensus-Based Entity (CBE), and in various measure evaluation and endorsement roles for the current CBE, the Battelle Partnership for Quality Measurement.

We thank Lauren Cowles from Cambridge University Press for having the patience of a saint! We are deeply indebted to Haley Abing, Harvard Medical School, for patiently and compulsively organizing the material in the book and keeping the project moving forward – she is an unsung hero without whom this book would not have been possible. We thank Mass-DAC staff (Ann Lovett, Tracey Silbaugh, Robert Wolf, Matt Cioffi, and Haley Abing), the cardiac surgeons, coronary interventionalists, and data managers in Massachusetts who adjudicated medical records, participated in numerous meetings, shared their insights, and from whom we learned invaluable lessons regarding the practical realities of quality measurement and public reporting.

Sharon-Lise Normand is grateful for her longstanding collaboration with Harlan Krumholz, Yale University, a cardiologist and leader in hospital quality assessments, and Yun Wang who, along with Harlan Krumholz and herself, implemented the hierarchical models for profiling the nation's cardiovascular hospital outcomes; and for early work with Constantine Gatsonis, Brown University, who introduced her to the statistical problem of profiling. David Shahian is thankful for his many colleagues in the Massachusetts General Hospital's Department of Surgery and Division of Cardiac Surgery; his longstanding measure development collaboration with Dr. Sean O'Brien of the Duke Clinical Research Institute; his quality measurement and research activities with Dr. Robert Habib, Jane Han, and many members of the STS quality and database staffs; his superb research manager and analyst Xiu Liu; and the hundreds of cardiac surgeons who have worked with him to measure, report, and improve cardiac surgery quality. Finally, we both greatly appreciate the abiding support and encouragement of our families, as well as our colleagues and students from whom we have learned so much.

CHAPTER EIGHTEEN

Preliminaries

We assume that the hierarchical structure of the data has two levels: level I units (e.g., patients and doctors) are clustered within level II units (e.g., hospitals and health plans). Definitions and assumptions are easily extended to settings in which there are more than two levels. Throughout, the *experimental unit* refers to level II units. Level I outcomes may include process measures, such as the appropriate use of beta blocker therapy, as well as outcome measures, such as survival. Selecting the basic components for comparison of healthcare quality across providers involves a number of key considerations as described in Table 18.1. We discuss these considerations in Sections 18.1–18.5.

18.1 Identifying the Study Population

After selecting a study population, for example, all Massachusetts hospitals treating adults undergoing Coronary artery bypass grafting (CABG) surgery, a process for determining how level I and II units will be identified from data is required. If working with billing claims data, then the sensitivity and specificity of the algorithm for inclusion of level I units and the algorithm for attributing level I units to level II units need to be considered. Identification of level I units involves both the inclusion of all units having the relevant condition or undergoing the particular procedure and the exclusion of level I units that do not meet the specification criteria for that condition. For example, if the goal is to study isolated CABG surgery, inclusion criteria must be specific enough to capture all such cases while excluding those cases in which CABG is combined with another major cardiac procedure, such as heart valve replacement. The latter cases have higher expected mortality rates, and their inclusion in a report of putative isolated CABG cases would produce misleading results. An example of this problem, reported by Shahian et al. [1], demonstrated how Massachusetts' report cards based on clinical and administrative data produced different results. Thus, the validity of the algorithm for identifying level I units often depends on the level of detail and quality of the data source used to select level I units.

The link between level I and II units needs to be conceptually sensible and clearly defined. Are all level I units clustered within level II units? While attribution of patients having an acute care admission to a hospital appears straightforward,

Table 18.1 Key considerations.

	Consideration	Example
1.	Study population	All hospitals in Massachusetts treating patients admitted with a heart attack; all US ambulatory care centers treating heart failure patients
2.	Policy target	How each hospital did with the patients it treated; how hospital *i* did compared to hospital *j*; how all hospitals treating a common set of patients performed (see Volume 2, Chapter 19, "A Causal Inference Framework")
3.	Level I outcomes	Cause-specific mortality; time to readmission; antibiotic use within 4 hours of hospital arrival (see Volume 1, Chapter 4, "Types of Performance Measures")
4.	Level II observational period of assessment	All hospital admissions within one year; all subjects treated by the health plan over a two-year period
5.	Data sources, risk factors, and confounders	Administrative billing data; survey data; registry data; medical record data (see Volume 1, Chapter 5, "Data Sources for Healthcare Quality Measurement")

patients can be transferred among hospitals. Should the patient be attributed to the first hospital or to the transfer hospital? A reasonable case could be made for either option. The decision between these two alternatives depends on the investigator's question. If the major focus of interest is characterization of level II outcomes to assess patients, overall treatment trajectories, then assignment to the index hospitalization makes sense. If interest rests on characterizing level II outcomes related to a particular event, such as surgery, then the hospital in which the surgery was performed may be the more relevant level II unit.

Attribution of level I units to level II units can quickly become complicated. When assessing the quality of outpatient care for heart failure patients, attributing patients to a unique outpatient provider (e.g., a level II unit) may be more difficult. Are level I units uniquely clustered within level II units, are level I units *partially clustered* within level II units, or is there no clustering of level I units within level II units? Some authors have used a *majority rule* assignment where patients are assigned to the ambulatory center where the majority of care was received. In many applications, the units at level I may themselves be structured by a cross-classification. For example, patients may be cross-classified by the hospital at which they were treated and the neighborhood in which they live. Interest may be centered on describing the variation between the hospital-neighborhood units. A simple extension to the labeling of the units [2] can be used to accommodate this setting, and we describe this further in Volume 2, Chapter 20, "Introduction to Hierarchical Linear Models."

Table 18.2 CABG surgery admissions. Commonwealth of Massachusetts, October 1, 2005–September 30, 2006.

Procedure type	Number of discharges	In-hospital mortality (%)	30-day mortality (%)
Isolated CABG	3684	1.41	1.41
Mitral valve replacement & CABG	67	5.97	7.46
Aortic valve replacement & CABG	514	3.70	4.47
CABG & other	628	7.96	7.17
Any procedure involving CABG	4893	2.48	2.64

18.1.1 Example: Hospital Mortality Following CABG Surgery

Table 18.2 lists the total number of hospital discharges for patients undergoing isolated CABG surgery (n = 3,684) and for patients having CABG surgery in addition to other major heart surgery, in the Commonwealth of Massachusetts during the period October 1, 2005, through September 30, 2006. Isolated CABG surgery refers to a surgical procedure in which CABG is the only major heart surgery performed. The table reports all-cause in-hospital (ranging from 1.41% to 7.96%) and 30-day mortality (ranging from 1.41% to 7.46%) stratified by type of heart surgery. Note that in-hospital mortality could be larger than 30-day mortality if the length of stay is longer than 30 days for some patients. This is likely the explanation for the "Other & CABG" procedures that include complex cases who had very prolonged hospitalizations, exceeding 30 days and died in the hospital after 30 days without ever having been discharged.

Which patient population should serve as the level I units in an assessment of the quality of hospital cardiac surgery? Examination of the mortality rates indicates differences in mortality risk across the various surgical procedure types, ranging from a low of 1.41% for isolated CABG surgery to a high of 7.96% for CABG in combination with surgical procedures other than valve replacement. Will the association between presenting patient risk factors and mortality differ depending on the procedure? Will the between-level II variation depend on the type of surgery? Are special surgical teams utilized for the different procedures so that hospital quality for one type of procedure could differ from its quality for another type of surgical procedure? The experimental unit, the relationship between risk factors and outcome, and the number of events and number of level I units will inform that decision.

18.2 Defining the Policy Targets

Historically, profiling activities have assessed hospital performance for the patients treated at the hospital. The policy target in this case is the specific hospital *conditional* on its associated patient case-mix. This task requires knowing what the outcomes of the patients treated at the hospital would have been had they been treated elsewhere. These unknown outcomes are denoted *counterfactual* or *potential* as they refer to what would have happened counter to the fact and must be estimated. Alternatively, a health plan may be interested in contracting with a set of hospitals and wants to know the quality of each hospital in the set of hospitals. The policy target is hospital quality for a randomly selected patient who could have been admitted to any of the hospitals under contract. If, for instance, one of the hospitals specializes in treating highly complex cases that differ from those of the other hospitals, these patients should not contribute to any estimates because such patients would not be treated at the other hospitals. Because a patient is treated at exactly one hospital, the counterfactual outcomes are those that would have occurred had the patient been treated at each of the other hospitals.

In both these examples, some method of estimating the counterfactual outcomes is required. Volume 1, Chapter 8, "Risk Modeling and Validation," described regression-based approaches to determining the counterfactual outcomes to assess hospital quality for the patients it treated, and we generally focus on this approach. Volume 2, Chapter 19, "A Causal Inference Framework," describes a causal inference framework for estimating counterfactual outcomes beyond regression-based approaches and for different policy targets.

18.3 Choosing Level I Outcomes

18.3.1 Fixed Follow-Up Time

The simplest type of outcome is one where all subjects are potentially observable for the same fixed period of time, such as receipt by heart attack patients of beta-blockade at hospital arrival or 30-day mortality following CABG surgery. In these examples, the outcome is binary and there are two possible types of responses—the patient does or does not receive the indicated medication, or the patient is either alive or dead at 30 days.

The binary probability model consists of Y failures out of N trials (or subjects) assuming that the probability of failure and of success is the sum of the individual probabilities. Two key assumptions of the binary probability model include: (1) the N trials are independent and (2) the failure rate is constant over the follow-up time. This implies that the probability of failure, p, for each subject is the same. If examining 30-day mortality, then we assume that the mortality rate within the first 15 days is the same as the mortality rate over days 16–30 (an assumption that may not hold for some situations with time-dependent hazard for mortality). Under these conditions, $Y_j \overset{\text{iid}}{\sim}$ Binomial (p, N), where the expected number of mortalities is Np, the variance is $Np(1 - p)$, and *iid* means independent and identically distributed. The level I outcome is therefore a binary-valued variable, Y_j, assuming a value of 0 or 1. Referring to the example presented in Table 18.2, the mortality risk appears constant between the in-hospital and 30-day time periods for isolated CABG surgery patients but seems to increase for admissions involving procedures additional to CABG surgery.

It is unlikely that the failure rate is identically distributed across patients in the observational setting. Rather, the probability of failure depends on patient-specific risk factors, x_j, so that the probability is denoted as $p(x_j)$, and some adjustment for observed risk factors is necessary. Moreover, because outcomes are hierarchically structured, even when assuming the mortality rate is constant over small time intervals, the assumptions of both independent trials (independence between level I units when clustered within a level II unit) and a constant failure probability (risk of dying is the same across Level II units) are violated. Probability distributions for accommodating hierarchical binary data are discussed in Volume 2, Chapter 21, "Hierarchical Generalized Linear Models."

18.3.2 Use of Exact Follow-Up Time

If the outcome is time to an event, such as hospital readmission within 30 days of a discharge, there are three possible types of responses—readmitted within 30 days of a discharge, died without a readmission, or no readmission for those surviving to 30 days. In this case, survival is a *censored* event (see Box 18.1) and death prior to a hospital readmission is a *competing* risk. Censoring refers to observations when no event or no competing risk is observed at the completion of follow-up; a subject has been censored at time t if she has been followed up to time t and has not failed. A competing risk is an event that prevents the occurrence of the primary outcome which is death in the example. Premature study termination for all other reasons, such as subject migration (the patient moves away from the study location), study withdrawal, or other reasons causing loss to follow-up are missing data. While missing data are often censored, this should not be the default strategy. For example, we would not expect censoring due to migration to introduce bias into provider comparisons. In contrast, if subjects withdraw from the study because of the quality of health care they received, then this may bias the results. Censoring is *non-informative* if the censored subjects have the same underlying survival curve after their censoring time as subjects who are not censored.

The treatment of censored outcomes involves modeling the failure *times* of individual subjects rather than the *occurrence* of the failure. In a setting where the incidence rates vary substantially over time, researchers typically focus on estimating the *survival function* $S(t)$, a function that yields the probability of survival up to time t for each $t \geqslant 0$. Suppose subjects are assessed at time $t_1, t_2, \cdots, t_m$, and interest centers on estimating survival up to time t_k (denoted $S(t_k)$) given the subject has survived up to time t_{k-1}. Assume S_k subjects are alive at t_k, d_k died, and l_k are censored. Then an estimate of survival at time t_k is as follows:

$$\hat{S}(t_k) = \left(1 - \frac{d_1}{S_0}\right) \times \left(1 - \frac{d_2}{S_1}\right) \times \cdots \times \left(1 - \frac{d_k}{S_{k-1}}\right). \tag{18.1}$$

The quantity in Eq. (18.1) is the product-limit (or Kaplan–Meier) estimator of survival in the presence of censored data. The failure rate (or hazard rate), $h(t)$, is estimated by

Box 18.1 Independent censoring

A censoring scheme is independent if the probability of censoring at each time t depends only on the observed covariates, the observed pattern of failures, and censoring information up to time t in the study, or on random processes that are independent of the failure times in the study.

$$h(t) = \left\{ \frac{S(t) - S(t + \Delta t)}{\Delta t} \right\} \times \frac{1}{S(t)},$$

as Δt approaches 0. The assumptions made in using the product-limit estimator are that censoring is non-informative and the observed survival times are independent. In the observational setting, survival times often depend on patient risk factors. However, when the outcomes are clustered, the assumption of independence is violated.

By far, the majority of quality measures are binary, and these outcome types will be used most frequently throughout the book.

18.3.3 Guidelines for Selecting Level I Outcomes

Volume 1, Chapter 4, "Types of Performance Measures," described a broad array of measure types available for healthcare quality measurement. Deciding which conditions and procedures would benefit the most from measurement, and which types of measures would be most appropriate, can be challenging. The National Quality Forum, an organization that, for several decades, was the legislatively designated Consensus-Based Entity (CBE) responsible for prioritizing and endorsing healthcare performance measures used by the Centers for Medicare & Medicaid Services (CMS), has provided recommendations to assist in evaluating these metrics and determining their suitability for accountability applications [3]. These include the following:

1. Importance to measure and report: a systematic assessment of the evidence base for the measure, and its potential to improve healthcare quality because of excessive variation in or suboptimal overall performance.
2. Scientific acceptability of measure properties: assure measure reliability and validity, as in similar measure guideline recommendations by the American College of Cardiology and the American Heart Association [4, 5].
3. Feasibility: the data are available and can be accurately and completely collected without excessive burden or cost.
4. Usability and use: stakeholders use or could use the results for accountability, transparency, and improvement of healthcare performance.
5. Competing or related measures: avoid duplication with closely related measures, harmonizing whenever possible.

Quite similar endorsement criteria are applied today by the current CBE, the Battelle Partnership for Quality Measurement [6–9]. The US federal government (e.g., the CMS Meaningful Measures initiative) and public–private partnerships, such as the Measure Applications Partnership, also provide continuing guidance in selection and prioritization of healthcare quality measures.

18.3.4 Example: CABG Surgery Outcomes

Most outcomes profiling initiatives for CABG patients include data on postoperative deaths and complications. However, there is considerable variability in the time frame during which such adverse outcomes are collected. Differences among institutional mortality rates resulting from non-standardized time intervals may be substantial [10]. For CABG surgery, there are three typical level I outcomes.

18.3.4.1 Fixed Follow-up Time

Common periods include 30-day mortality following a surgical procedure and readmission within 30 days of a discharge. Thirty-day mortality, for example, means that all deaths occurring within 30 days of surgery are recorded, regardless of venue. Thirty-day follow-up is costly and difficult to obtain because it requires follow-up with the patient. Even with a fixed follow-up period, there is still an opportunity to game the system (Volume 1, Chapter 15, "Unintended Consequences") by keeping alive, terminally ill patients just long enough to pass the 30-day endpoint.

Advances in critical care have resulted in the prolonged survival of some patients who previously would have died in the early postoperative period. This includes patients who may spend prolonged periods in chronic care facilities on dialysis or mechanical ventilation. Such considerations have led some to argue that the definition of the early postoperative period should be lengthened considerably, perhaps to as long as 180 days [11]. Linkages to administrative data sources make even longer follow-up periods (e.g., years) possible. However, from a profiling perspective, the direct association between quality of care and outcomes may be progressively confounded by exogenous factors the longer the interval between treatment and follow-up.

18.3.4.2 In-hospital Mortality and Morbidity

This is the only approach available from many data sources, and it was used in the original CABG mortality analyses from New York state [12]. The primary advantages are cost and practicality—these data are readily available and require no additional effort at some later time following discharge. Proponents argue that most post-procedural deaths occur during the index hospitalization and that the difference between in-hospital and 30-day mortality is small. Furthermore, in-hospital deaths are most proximate to, and theoretically most likely to have a causal association with, the quality of care that was administered. Conversely, there are distinct disadvantages to limiting data collection to the in-hospital period. First, there is the possibility of intentional gaming, as first recognized by Florence Nightingale 150 years ago. Anticipating an adverse outcome, a hospital could transfer a patient to another institution or extended care facility, where the patient's subsequent mortality is either unreported or attributed to the wrong facility. Second, hospitals vary in their ability to transfer patients to such extended care facilities. Thus, some institutions must keep patients hospitalized for longer periods postoperatively, with a correspondingly greater chance that adverse events will occur and be recorded during the index admission. Some hospitals with a network of extended care facilities have a greater ability to transfer patients earlier in their postoperative course, with consequently reduced exposure for the original institution. Recording only in-hospital mortality may thus differentially disadvantage some providers [13], a form of ascertainment bias. Another concern is that pressures have increased for early discharge of patients. Some complications, like sternal infection, may not become clinically relevant in a short hospital stay and may present after hospital discharge. The subsequent readmission for treatment of this infection may be missed in some data registries, particularly if the patient goes to a different institution. In some instances, complications and readmissions (delayed complications) may reflect different aspects of care than mortality, and it is important to capture both whenever possible [14, 15]. A serious complication may result in death at one institution because of failure to rescue, whereas better care for a similar complication at another institution may result in patient survival.

18.3.4.3 Combined Approaches

This approach attempts to capture all early deaths related to surgery, at the expense of having a potentially nonstandardized follow-up period. It is used by the Society of Thoracic Surgeons (where it is referred to as Operative Mortality) and by the New York State Cardiac Surgery Reporting System. The idea is to capture all early deaths related to surgery, at the expense of having a potentially nonstandardized follow-up period. All deaths occurring in-hospital during the index admission are recorded, regardless of timing, as are all deaths occurring within 30 days of surgery, regardless of venue. This maximizes the likelihood of capturing all procedure-related deaths and minimizes the gaming opportunity. However, ascertainment bias is introduced because the follow-up period is not fixed across patients.

As demonstrated here, more than one level I outcome may be of importance. Typically, the multiple outcomes are modeled separately or combined into a composite measure (Volume 1, Chapter 11, "Composite Performance Measures"). Modeling outcomes separately has several limitations and statistical approaches for joint modeling of multiple outcomes are discussed in Volume 2, Chapter 22, "Composite Measures and Multiple Outcomes."

18.4 Determining the Level II Observational Period

Determining the appropriate time frame during which to collect information on level II units is a function of several factors. A major consideration is whether the level II outcomes are constant. If the goal is to estimate the quality of a provider, then it is desirable to have the performance constant across the observational period. If there are interventions to improve processes of care or outcomes over the observational period, then those improvements may be masked. However, the outcome rate and the number of both level I and II units impact the accuracy of the level II effects. For example, if a minimum of 400 patients (level I units) are needed to reliably estimate risk-standardized mortality for each cardiac surgeon (level II units), it may only be feasible to accrue that number of level I units if all surgeries performed by cardiac surgeons over three years are collected. The assumption in this instance is that cardiac surgeon performance is approximately constant across the three-year observational period.

18.4.1 Example: Outcome Measures for Heart Attacks and CABG Surgery

Tables 18.3a and 18.3b give examples of the provider sample sizes over different observational periods, different level II units, and different measures for two US states, California and Massachusetts, and for two study populations: hospital quality for heart attack victims (Table 18.3a) and CABG surgery mortality for hospitals

Table 18.3a Publicly reported outcomes (heart attack).

State	Level II Unit	Measure	No. of units (% of total units)	Mean number patients per unit	Obs. period (months)
CA	Hospital[a]	In-hospital ASA	350 (95)	10	8
		Discharge ACEI	208 (57)	3	8
		Discharge β-blocker	298 (81)	6	8
		Discharge ASA	328 (89)	8	8
MA		In-Hospital ASA	80 (99)	21	8
		Discharge ACEI	73 (90)	5	8
		Discharge β-blocker	80 (99)	11	8
		Discharge ASA	80 (99)	16	8

ASA, aspirin; ACEI, angiotensin-converting enzyme inhibitor. Heart attack measures taken from Normand et al. (2007) [16] based on data collected between February 1994 and July 1995 as part of the Cooperative Cardiovascular Project initiated by HCFA.

[a]All hospitals are nonfederal general/medical or specialty "heart hospitals" that focus on cardiovascular care. Inclusion criteria for hospitals differ for each measure, but each measure is restricted to Medicare patients aged 65 to 89. Patients hospitalized between February 1994 and July 1995.

Table 18.3b Publicly reported outcomes (isolated CABG surgery).

State	Level II Unit	Measure	No. of units (% of total units)	Mean number patients per unit	Obs. period (years)
CA	Hospital[a]	Mortality	121 (100)	159.2	1
MA		Mortality	14 (100)	284.7	1
CA	Surgeon[b]	Mortality	278 (92)	144.9	2
MA		Mortality	56 (98)	218.8	3

CABG, coronary artery bypass grafting. CABG surgery hospital and surgeon numbers are reported publicly on state-specific websites.

[a]Includes all nonfederal acute care hospitals in the state that treated at least one isolated CABG surgery patient. Patients are aged 18 years or older. Data are for surgeries performed between January 1, 2004, and December 31, 2004.

[b]Includes surgeons who treated at least 10 isolated CABG surgery patients across all hospitals and years. Patients are aged 18 years or older. California data use surgeries performed between January 1, 2003, and December 31, 2004 (see www.oshpd.ca.gov); Massachusetts data use surgeries performed between January 1, 2003, and December 31, 2005.

and surgeons (Table 18.3b). The two states differ in many ways that together result in different sample sizes on which to base quality estimates. California has a much larger population compared to Massachusetts—36 million residents compared to 6 million residents. The number of acute care hospitals in California is more than four times that in Massachusetts (357 hospitals vs. 81 hospitals). The number of hospital admissions is lower in California (95 per 1000 residents) compared to that in Massachusetts (130 admissions per 1000 residents). Finally, the number of deaths due to diseases of the heart is higher in California (196 per 100,000 population) than that in Massachusetts (173 per 100,000 population).

The data in Tables 18.3a,b are derived from several sources. Table 18.3a reports on the process of care measures for patients treated for a heart attack and includes the use of aspirin during the hospitalization, and three discharge medications: angiotensin-converting enzyme inhibitors (ACEI), beta-blocker, and aspirin. The processes of care measures are derived from clinical data collected between February 1994 and July 1995 for a cohort of Medicare patients aged 65 to 89 years in the two states. During this time frame, 368 CA hospitals and 81 MA hospitals treated at least one Medicare patient discharged with a heart attack in an eight-month sampling period. Because of specific contraindications, not all heart attack patients are ideal candidates for the specific process measurements. For example, in determining the number of Medicare patients eligible for ACEI at discharge, the following patients are excluded if coded as having: a *do not resuscitate* order on day 1, terminal illness, left ventricular ejection fraction >40%, died during hospitalization, aortic stenosis, ACEI allergy, serum creatinine >2 mg/dL, and systolic blood pressure <100 mmHg at discharge. Table 18.3b reports on mortality outcomes following CABG surgery for those aged 18 years or greater at the time of the surgery during 2004 for hospitals; between 2003 and 2004 for CA surgeons and between January 1, 2003, and December 31, 2005 for MA surgeons.

18.5 Risk Factors and Confounders

Risk factors typically refer to variables that change or impact the occurrence of the outcome, whereas confounders are variables that impact both the outcome and provider choice. Risk factors and confounders are not mutually exclusive. If sicker patients are more likely to undergo surgery at a specialty cardiac hospital and sicker patients have a higher chance of not surviving, then patient "sickness" is a confounder. If hospitals have the same age distribution of the patients they treat, then age is a risk factor (rather than a confounder) for mortality. Risk factors may be important to include in analyses to increase the precision of the treatment effect [17]; however, they are not necessary to include. Confounders must be included to draw valid inferences.

As described in Volume 1, Chapter 8, "Risk Modeling and Validation," only those features present at the time the patient begins the episode of care for which performance is being monitored (e.g., an admission for acute myocardial infarction or major surgery) should be considered for inclusion in the risk model. It would be inappropriate to include events, characteristics, or risk factors that occurred or first developed after admission and before the specific endpoint because they are on the *causal pathway*. Post-admission risk factors are likely predictive of the final outcome, they may have resulted from inadequate care by the provider, and consequently, they should not be "adjusted out" through modeling. For instance, adjustment of a mortality performance measure for infections occurring during treatment would be inappropriate. The infection might increase the risk of mortality, but it may have resulted from poor sterilization or infection control practices by the provider. Effectively, patients who develop infections during their hospitalizations would then be treated similarly to those who present with a significant infectious comorbidity, such as pneumonia or sepsis. The conflation of comorbidities and complications has historically been one of the most serious issues with provider profiling based on claims data. Present on admission indicators and a one-year look-back at prior visits or hospitalizations are two mechanisms used to mitigate this problem [18].

18.6 Summary

The basic building blocks for measuring provider quality, while seemingly simple, often lack clarity. The specification of the study population, the target policy, and how the patients (level I) are assigned to providers (level II) are required to yield meaningful assessments. Level I outcomes could be univariate (single outcomes) or multivariate (multiple outcomes) and likely have different probability distributions. The period of provider assessment varies with the study population and the endpoint. The process of estimation of counterfactual outcomes requires risk adjustment and is the subject of the next Chapter 19.

CHAPTER NINETEEN

A Causal Inference Framework

Discussions of the concept of causation date to antiquity and are found in a variety of disciplines, including philosophy (e.g., Aristotle, Hume, Mill), logic, mathematics, statistics, and computer science [19–23]. Viewed from the most simplistic perspective, an exposure or intervention is causative if, in its absence, the subsequent event would not have occurred. The nuances of causation theory are beyond the scope of this book, and the interested reader is encouraged to consult the works of Pearl [24], Rothman and Greenland [21], and the comprehensive work led by Rubin referenced in this chapter.

The difference between what happened to the individual, given a specific exposure or intervention, and what would have happened under another set of circumstances (e.g., absent the intervention) is a measure of the *causal effect* of that intervention. Early examples reflect the state of scientific knowledge in those eras. For example, because of the agrarian nature of economies in the 17th and 18th centuries, causal thinking was often applied to common agricultural questions, such as comparing the crop yield from one type of seeding or fertilization with another [23]. In medicine, Koch's postulates for microbial disease were introduced during the late 19th century and reflect a causal association approach.

The formal application of causal theory to scientific experimentation began in the early 20th century. The Polish Statistician Neyman and the English Statistician Fisher introduced the concept of randomization as a useful approach to rigorously determining causal effects [22, 23]. In his classic 1965 publication, the English statistician and epidemiologist Sir Austin Bradford Hill (who with colleague Richard Doll had demonstrated the link between smoking and lung cancer) elucidated nine principles to be used when attempting to separate true causation from mere association [25]. It was not until the last decades of the 20th century that the statistical concepts of causal inference were fully developed and generalized to non-randomized, observational studies by a number of prominent researchers, including Rubin, Robins, Pearl, Greenland, Rothman, Holland, Rosenbaum, and others [19–24, 26–34]. In this book, we use Rosenbaum's [31] definition of an observational study as one that "concerns treatments, interventions, or policies, and the effects they cause."

In this chapter, we begin by casting the profiling problem as a causal inference problem, using Rubin's framework. The causal parameters that are often policy targets are listed, and key assumptions required to make valid statistical inferences are described in Sections 19.1–19.4. Several estimators that rely on parametric modeling are characterized. We conclude the chapter with a discussion of two more recent topics: machine learning approaches in general and approaches that constrain the distribution of the risk factors directly.

19.1 The Rubin Causal Model

One important and widely accepted framework for studying causal inference is the Rubin Causal Model [22, 23, 29, 35–39]. The goal of this model is to systematize the determination of the causal parameter that we want to estimate. The causal effect is defined as a function (e.g., a difference or ratio) of the observed outcome and the outcome in the absence of the intervention for an *individual*. The fundamental problem of causal inference, as described by Holland in 1986 [19], is that only one outcome is observable for each individual at a given time—namely, the result of the actual exposure experienced by the individual. For instance, a patient cannot simultaneously undergo different operations or undergo the same operation at different hospitals at the same time. One operation and its outcome are observed, while the outcome associated with the other operation is missing. The missing outcome is referred to as the *potential or counterfactual outcome*. As this outcome is unobservable, it must be estimated, and therein lies one of the most critical problems faced by outcomes researchers.

In healthcare profiling, many different possible policy targets lead to different causal parameters. Let Y_{ij} denote the observed outcome for patient j assigned to provider i; $H_{ij} = 1$ if patient j is treated by provider i and 0 otherwise; and let $Y_{ij}(H_{ij})$ denote the potential outcome, that is, the outcome had patient j been treated by provider i. The outcomes are *potential* because, in theory, any patient could be treated by any provider, and we therefore could potentially observe the outcome. Under some specific assumptions discussed next, the observed outcome is represented as

$$Y_{ij} = H_{1j}Y_{1j}(H_{1j}) + H_{2j}Y_{2j}(H_{2j}) + \cdots + H_{ij}Y_{ij}(H_{ij}) + \cdots + H_{Ij}Y_{Ij}(H_{Ij}), \quad (19.1)$$

where I is the total number of providers.[1] Here providers are treatments, and the goal is to estimate the effect of provider i on patient outcomes. The "treatments" can be manipulated: we could close the hospital, restrict the types of patients treated by a provider, or make other policy changes.

The formulation in Eq. 19.1 relates to the notion of *multivalued* treatments where patients, in theory, could be treated by any of the hospitals.[2]

19.2 Causal Effect

As a specific example, suppose there are only two providers and a patient could undergo CABG surgery at either one. The observed outcome can be written as

[1] Some authors use different notation, ignoring the clustered nature of the data. Let A_j assume values $1, 2, \ldots, I$ and let $(A_j = i) = 1$ if patient j was treated at hospital i and 0 otherwise. Then, $Y_j(A_j = i)$ denotes the counterfactual outcome for patient j when treated at hospital i.

[2] The counterfactual outcomes obtained here are like those obtained via direct standardization.

$$Y_{ij} = H_{1j} Y_{1j}(H_{1j}) + H_{2j} Y_{2j}(H_{2j}).$$

There are two possible outcomes for individual j: $Y_{1j}(H_{1j})$, the outcome if patient j was treated by provider 1 and $Y_{2j}(H_{2j})$, the outcome if treated by provider 2. The causal effect could be defined as

$$\delta_j = Y_{1j}(H_{1j}) - Y_{2j}(H_{2j}). \tag{19.2}$$

Alternatively, the causal effect could be defined as the ratio of the two potential outcomes, $Y_{1j}(H_{1j})/Y_{2j}(H_{2j})$.

19.3 Causal Parameter

A causal parameter is the average of person-level causal effects. Returning to the two provider examples, the causal parameter is defined as the average of the individual causal effects,

$$\delta_{\text{ATE}} = \frac{1}{N}\sum_{j*=1}^{N}\left\{Y_{1j*}(H_{1j*}) - Y_{2j*}(H_{2j*})\right\} \text{ where } N = n_1 + n_2 \tag{19.3}$$

and n_i is the number of patients treated by the ith provider. The average is taken over all patients, and so we use the index $j*$. The parameter δ_{ATE} is denoted the "average treatment effect (ATE)." More specifically, we are concerned with the *sample average treatment effects* (SATE) as it is the average of the individual treatment effects over a finite sample but we will generally drop the "S." The population average treatment effect (PATE) is defined as $\mathbb{E}(Y(H_1) - Y(H_2))$.

In earlier examples, a different policy target involved determining the average effect *among those treated* by provider 1, which is defined as

$$\delta_{\text{ATT}} = \frac{1}{n_1}\sum_{j=1}^{n_1}\left\{Y_{1j}(H_{1j}) - Y_{2j}(H_{2j}) \mid H_{1j} = 1\right\}. \tag{19.4}$$

The | symbol implies *conditional on*. The parameter, δ_{ATT}, is called the "average treatment effect among the treated (ATT)," which characterizes the provider effect for patients treated by provider 1. This may differ from the ATE if provider 2 treats some patients that differ from those treated by provider 1.

Causal effects among patient subgroups may also be of interest. For example, a patient with diabetes needing CABG surgery may be interested in determining whether she should select hospital 1 or 2. This causal parameter is

$$\delta_{\text{CATE}}(x) = \frac{1}{n(x)}\sum_{j:X=x}^{n(x)}\left\{Y_{1j}(H_{1j}) - Y_{2j}(H_{2j})\right\}, \tag{19.5}$$

where $n(x)$ is the number of patients with covariate value x = diabetes. The causal parameter $\delta(x)$ is denoted the "conditional average treatment effect (CATE)" given it refers to causal effects among a subpopulation conditional on or characterized by the covariate x.

Table 19.1 Causal parameters for policy targets. We drop the S from SATE and SATT.

Target parameter	Population
Sample average treatment Effect (δ_{ATE})	Patients selected from all providers
Sample average treatment Effect among the treated (δ_{ATT})	Patients selected from the specific provider
Conditional average treatment effect ($\delta_{\text{CATE}}(X)$)	Patients with covariate value, $X = x$, sampled from all providers
Conditional average treatment effect among the treated ($\delta_{\text{CATT}}(X)$)	Patients with covariate value, $X = x$, sampled from the specific provider

With many providers, many causal parameters are possible, and the specific choice depends on the policy target (see Table 19.1). For instance, the ATT is

$$\delta_{\text{ATT},i} = \frac{1}{n_i}\sum_{j=1}^{n_i}\left\{ Y_{ij}(H_{ij}) - Y_{i^*j}(H_{i^*j}) \mid H_{ij} = i\right\}, \quad (19.6)$$

where $i^* \neq i$ refers to all providers except provider i. The parameter in Eq. 19.6 represents the effect of provider i on the outcome for *a randomly sampled patient treated by provider i* compared to receiving care from a provider other than i. Alternatively, interest may center on determining whether that care received at provider i differs from the care the patient could have received if treated by a specific provider, k.

19.4 Assumptions

Let $N = \sum_{i=1}^{I} n_i$, I the number of providers, $\mathbf{H}_i = N \times 1$ vector with ith element H_{ij}, $\mathbf{X} = N \times p$ matrix of confounders, and $\mathbf{Y}(H_i) = N \times 1$ vector of potential outcomes for individuals treated by provider i, noting that each individual has I potential outcomes of which exactly one is observed. We let $\mathbf{X}_{ij}$ denote a $1 \times p$ vector of covariates for the jth patient treated by the ith provider, and denote the kth element of $\mathbf{X}_{ij}$ by X_{kij}. The set of assumptions required to infer causal effects is next described.

19.4.1 The SUTVA

The stable unit treatment assumption (SUTVA) enables the expression of the observed outcome as

$$Y_{ij} = H_{1j}Y_{1j}(H_{1j}) + H_{2j}Y_{2j}(H_{2j}) + \cdots + H_{ij}Y_{ij}(H_{ij}) + \cdots + H_{Ij}Y_{Ij}(H_{Ij}) \quad (19.7)$$

and comprises two assumptions.

19.4.1.1 No Interference

No interference assumes that treatments applied to one subject do not affect the outcomes for another subject. A simple illustration, provided by Imbens and Rubin

[39], involves assessing the effectiveness of aspirin on the occurrence of a headache. No interference implies that if individual A takes an aspirin, that does not affect whether individual B gets a headache. This assumption seems reasonable. When assessing the quality of healthcare providers, no interference means that the quality of care delivered to individual A does not affect the outcome of individual B. This is sensible if individuals A and B are treated by *different* providers and there are no *spillover effects* on patients treated at different hospitals. How could this assumption be violated when assessing providers? Suppose we are assessing hospital cardiac surgical quality, and most of the cardiac surgeons at a large academic hospital 1 also moonlight at hospital 2. In this situation, patient postsurgical survival in hospital 2 may be better because procedural strategies originally employed by surgeons in hospital 1 are then also applied at hospital 2. The quality of care provided by a hospital will also be impacted by resources available at the hospital, such as nursing staff, ICU intensivist coverage, medical residents, and the number of cardiac surgeons unique to hospital 2. These resources may differ between the two hospitals, and the larger the differences, the weaker the spillover effects.

We *do* expect the provider's quality to affect the outcomes of other individuals treated by the *same* provider. Conditioning on other variables may remove this dependence.

19.4.1.2 No Hidden Variations of Treatments

This assumption requires "treatments" to be well-defined so that exposure to the treatment leads to a well-defined outcome or set of outcomes. In the earlier example, an aspirin is an aspirin – there is not much ambiguity there! When assessing the quality of healthcare providers, the treatment is the provider, which is typically well-defined. However, instances where assigning individuals to providers may not be straightforward were described in Volume 2, Chapter 18, "Preliminaries."

19.4.2 Assignment Mechanism

The algorithm used to assign patients to a provider is called the *assignment mechanism*. For each patient j, the assignment to provider i can be expressed as

$$
\begin{aligned}
q_{ij} &= p_{ij}(H_{ij} = 1 \mid \mathbf{X}_{ij}, Y_{1j}(H_{1j}), Y_{2j}(H_{2j}), \ldots, Y_{Ij}(H_{Ij})), \ \sum_{i=1}^{I} q_{ij} = 1 \\
&\overset{\text{SUTVA}}{=} p_{ij}(H_{ij} = 1 \mid \mathbf{X}_{ij}, Y_{ij}(H_{ij})). \qquad (19.8)
\end{aligned}
$$

The SUTVA enables the provider assignment for an individual to be independent of the provider assignment of other individuals and to only depend on the individual's covariates and potential outcomes. The probability of provider assignment for the sample is

$$
c \times \prod_{j=1}^{N} q_{1j}(\mathbf{X}_{1j}, Y_{1j}(H_{1j}))^{H_{1j}} q_{2j}(\mathbf{X}_{2j}, Y_{2j}(H_{2j}))^{H_{2j}} \cdots q_{Ij}(\mathbf{X}_{Ij}, Y_{Ij}(H_{Ij}))^{H_{Ij}}
$$

where c is a normalizing constant. If interested in the ATT_i, then the assignment mechanism is viewed as

$$c \times \prod_{j=1}^{N} q_{ij}(\mathbf{X}_{ij}, Y_{ij}(H_{ij}))^{H_{ij}}(1 - q_{ij}(\mathbf{X}_{ij}, Y_{ij}(H_{ij})))^{1-H_{ij}},$$

that is, there are only two choices: treated by provider i or not. Note that using this formulation for each provider separately does not guarantee $\sum_i^I q_{ij} = 1$.

19.4.2.1 Positivity

The positivity assumption presupposes that each individual has a nonzero chance of undergoing care from any of the providers,

$$0 < q_{ij} < 1 \text{ for all } i \ \& \ j. \tag{19.9}$$

This assumption may be violated in two ways. First, some patient subgroups may never be treated by a specific provider. Some states, for instance, restrict primary angioplasty, a type of coronary intervention for patients having a heart attack, to only hospitals having backup cardiac surgery. Thus, we will never observe hospitals without backup cardiac surgery providing primary angioplasty to patients having a heart attack. This is a *structural* positivity violation. Second, other violations may emerge simply because the sample is too small. For instance, cardiogenic shock is infrequent, and some hospitals in the sample may not have treated any patients arriving in cardiogenic shock. If the provider size was larger or the period of observation longer, then such patients are likely to have been observed at the provider. These violations are referred to as *finite sample size* positivity violations.

A violation of the positivity assumption means that there is a lack of *overlap* in the assignment mechanism, meaning there may be some regions of the covariate space that define patient subgroups where there are either no or very few patients from some providers. Estimates of provider quality for these patient subgroups will either be based entirely on extrapolation or be unstable. Panels A–D in Figure 19.1 display the probability of treatment at hospital 1, q_{1j}, for each of the 4 hospitals. In Panel A, the distribution of q_{1j} completely overlaps that of patients treated at hospital 2 (indicated by the dashed line). In Panel B, while q_{1j}s for patients treated at hospital 3 (dashed line) partially overlaps with q_{1j} among those treated at hospital 1, there are no patients in hospital 1 with assignment probabilities larger than 0.30 although there are patients treated at hospital 1 having such probabilities. Thus, there is only a small area of overlap in Panel B. In Panels A and B, the average probabilities of treatment in hospital 1 are generally similar for those patients treated in hospitals 1, 2, and 3. Panels C and D display situations in which the average probabilities of treatment at hospital 1 differ between those treated at hospital 1 and the other hospitals. In C, there is overlap across all probabilities for patients treated at hospitals 1 and 4, whereas in D, the overlap of probabilities is small between those treated at hospitals 1 and 5.

19.4.2.2 Unconfoundedness

The assignment mechanism is *unconfounded* if the assignment does not depend on the potential outcomes,

Figure 19.1 Overlap distributions for probability of treatment at hospital 1, q_{1j}. Solid line is density estimate for q_{1j} among those treated at hospital 1; dashed lines are density estimates for q_{1j} among those observed to be treated at different hospitals.

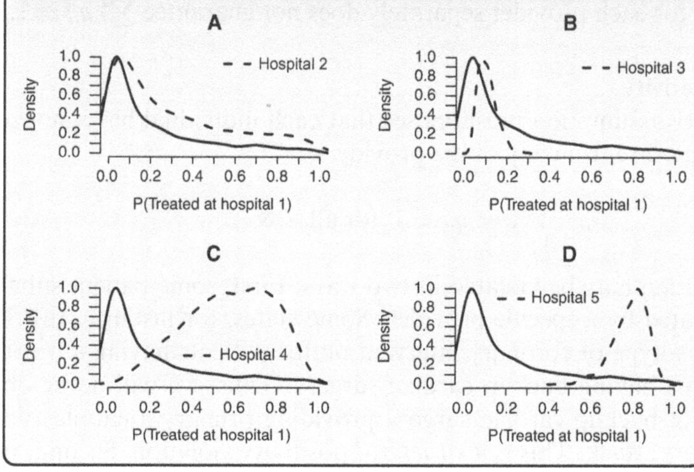

$$Pr(\mathbf{X}, \mathbf{Y}(\mathbf{H}_1), \mathbf{Y}(\mathbf{H}_2), \ldots, \mathbf{Y}(\mathbf{H}_J)) = Pr(\mathbf{X}, H, Y). \quad (19.10)$$

By far, the unconfoundedness assumption has received the most attention in assessing provider quality of care. For instance, in examining 30-day mortality following surgery across hospitals, patient complexity differs across hospitals, and complexity is certainly related to mortality. Including sufficiently rich covariates to ensure patient complexity is unconfounded with provider assignment is therefore a key goal in making inferences.

Often claims of unmeasured confounders are raised. However, unconfoundedness is not directly testable, so (1) investigators should demonstrate robustness of findings to unmeasured confounders and (2) those raising these concerns should provide information that supports these claims. Strategies to reduce the likelihood of unconfoundedness include a strong study design (e.g., randomization, prospective data collection), quality of data collection (e.g., standardized tool), type of data (see Volume 1, Chapter 5, "Data Sources for Healthcare Quality Measurement"), and the availability of measured confounders. Similarity in confounder distributions is referred to as *covariate balance*. An imbalance in the distribution of a confounder implies that some adjustment must be made to account for the differences in the confounder distributions. Approaches to assessing the unconfoundedness assumption exist and are discussed in Volume 2, Chapter 25, "Model Assessment."

19.4.3 Sample

A key premise often overlooked involves the selection of the sample to be used for inference. The units studied should be a sample from the target population so it is desirable to have some knowledge of the sample selection mechanism.[3] For instance, if the sample is drawn randomly from the study population so that positivity holds and, on average, unconfoundedness holds, then causal parameters such as the ATE or the ATT are identified. However, like randomized studies in which healthier rather than sicker patients typically participate, patients are unlikely to have been drawn randomly from the study population. In observational studies, for instance, patients included in a clinical registry may be representative of those treated at large, academic hospitals if smaller hospitals do not have the resources to create registries. Generalizability of the causal effects therefore depends on how representative the sample is of the study population.

The problem of assessing the generalizability of results to target populations has garnered attention from several disciplines. Approaches to translating randomized trial results to target populations using propensity scores have been proposed [41–44] as have methods that combine randomized studies with observational studies [45] and methods that combine heterogeneous data sources [46]. A clear understanding of how the sample arose is thus important in making statements about provider quality.

19.5 Estimators

Risk adjustment is the term commonly used to describe the analytical approach to balance confounders across providers when profiling (see Volume 1, Chapter 8, "Risk Modeling and Validation"). Historically this term incorrectly encompassed two statistical concepts: the selection of the policy target and the approach to balancing the confounders across providers. The two most frequent approaches in provider profiling to estimate the counterfactual outcomes are those defined through *direct* and *indirect* standardization [47] via regression modeling. However, approaches beyond outcome regression modeling, such as those that use the provider assignment mechanism only and those that use a combination of both approaches, are available.

There are two main causal parameters of interest:

$$\delta_{\mathrm{ATT},i} = = \frac{1}{n_1}\sum_{j=1}^{n_1}\left\{ Y_{ij}(H_{ij}=1) - Y_{ij}(H_{ij}=0) \mid H_{ij}=1 \right\}. \tag{19.11}$$

$\delta_{\mathrm{ATT},i}$ is the ATT causal parameter. The first term, $\frac{1}{n_1}\sum_{j=1}^{n_1}\left\{ Y_{ij}(H_{ij}=1)\right\}$, can be estimated by the observed mean.[4] It is the estimator of the counterfactual, $Y_{ij}(H_{ij}=0)$, that requires much more work. The other causal parameter is the ATE

$$\delta_i = \frac{1}{N}\sum_{j*=1}^{N}\left\{ Y_{ij*}(H_{ij*}=i) - Y_{ij*}(H_{ij*}=0)\right\} \tag{19.12}$$

that may also be of interest.

[3] Randomization-based inference [40] is another approach that assumes the sample is fixed and only the treatment assignment is random. In this framework, technically, the sample need not be thought of as a sample from some larger population.

[4] Small sample size issues and use of shrinkage estimators are discussed in Chapters 20 and 21.

19.5.1 Outcome Regression Modeling

Assume

$$m(X, \beta) = \frac{1}{n_1}\sum_{j=1}^{n_1}\left\{Y_{ij}(H_{ij}=0) \mid X_{ij}, H_{ij}=1\right\} = \frac{1}{n_1}\sum_{j=1}^{n_1}\left\{Y_{ij} \mid X_{ij}, H_{ij}=0, \beta\right\}.$$

The counterfactual outcome if individual i had been treated by a provider other than i conditional on the observed confounders can be estimated using a parametric regression model by pooling data across all providers except provider i. Because these estimates are regression-based, they are targeting the CATT. Plug-in estimates of β are used to get $m(X, \widehat{\beta})$ yielding

$$\widehat{\delta}_{\text{CATT},i} = \frac{1}{n_i}\sum_{j=1}^{n_i} Y_{ij} - \frac{1}{n_i}\sum_{j=1}^{n_i} m(X_{ij}, \widehat{\beta}). \tag{19.13}$$

Rather than differences, the causal parameter using indirect standardization is typically defined as a ratio of the observed outcome relative to the potential outcome (**Box 19.1**) for each provider. In earlier approaches implemented outside of a causal inference setting, patients from all providers are pooled, including those treated at $H_{ij}=1$, to obtain $\widehat{\beta}$, which is problematic.

Additional points are worth noting. Most researchers have used indirect standardization via parametric modeling to estimate the CATT. Parametric models are widely familiar; they produce parameters that are easily interpreted, such as odds ratios or relative risks, that users can examine; the models are typically parsimonious, making it easy to understand the influence of specific risk factors; and model fit can be assessed using standard approaches, all of which make the results transparent to users. The key issues are whether Y_i is a good estimator for $\frac{1}{n_i}\sum_{j=1}^{n_i} Y_{ij}(H_{ij})$ and $\widehat{p}_i$ is a good estimator for $\frac{1}{n_1}\sum_{j=1}^{n_1}\left\{Y_{ij}(H_{ij}=0) \mid X_{ij}, H_{ij}=1\right\}$.

Box 19.1 Indirect standardization: Observed to expected outcome (O/E)

Suppose Y_{ij} is a binary outcome for the jth subject treated by provider i such that

$$Y_{ij} \overset{ind}{\sim} \text{Bern}(p_{ij}(\mathbf{X})) \text{ where } \text{logit}(p_{ij}(\mathbf{X})) = \theta + \boldsymbol{\beta}'\mathbf{X}_{ij}.$$

The potential outcome for provider i is

$$p_i = \frac{1}{n_i}\sum_{j=1}^{n_i} p_{i,j}(\mathbf{X}) = \frac{1}{n_i}\sum_{j=1}^{n_i}\text{logit}^{-1}\left(\theta + \boldsymbol{\beta}'\mathbf{X}_{ij}\right) \tag{19.14}$$

and the observed outcome is $Y_i = \frac{1}{n_i}\sum_{j=1}^{n_i} Y_{ij}$. The estimator of the causal ratio for provider i is

$$\frac{Y_i}{\widehat{p}_i} \text{ where } \widehat{p}_i = \frac{1}{n_i}\sum_{j=1}^{n_i}\hat{p}_{ij} = \frac{1}{n_i}\sum_{j=1}^{n_i}\text{logit}^{-1}\left(\widehat{\theta} + \widehat{\boldsymbol{\beta}}'\mathbf{X}_{ij}\right). \tag{19.15}$$

Values larger than 1 indicate higher-than-expected outcomes (which would be worse when referring to an adverse outcome such as mortality) and values less than 1 indicate lower-than-expected outcomes (which would be better when referring to adverse outcomes).

Volume 2, Chapter 20, "Introduction to Hierarchical Linear Models," and Chapter 5, "Hierarchical Generalized Linear Models," will show these estimators may not be ideal.

What about direct standardization? In this setup, interest centers on the expected outcome had all patients been treated by provider i. The estimator for the ith provider is

$$\widehat{p}_i = \frac{1}{\sum_{s=1}^{I} n_i} \sum_{i}^{I} \sum_{j=1}^{n_i} \widehat{p}(X_{sj}) \text{ where } \widehat{p}(X_{sj}) = \text{logit}^{-1}\left(\widehat{\theta}_i + \widehat{\boldsymbol{\beta}}'\mathbf{X}_{sj}\right) \quad (19.16)$$

with θ_i a provider-specific effect. Note that the sum is taken over all patients and all providers. In this approach, meaningful differences across providers would signal provider variability in quality of care. This approach assumes that any patient could have been treated by any provider. This is often a heroic assumption.

More generally, assume that the potential outcome for a patient cared for by provider i is characterized using a generalized linear regression model, $m(X_{ij}, \theta_i, \boldsymbol{\beta})$, with link function l where

$$l(\mathbb{E}(Y_{ij}(H_{ij}) \mid \mathbf{X}_{ij})) = \theta_1 H_{1j} + \cdots + \theta_I H_{Ij} + \boldsymbol{\beta}'\mathbf{X}_{ij}. \quad (19.17)$$

Here, the potential outcome for each patient varies by an additive provider effect, θ_i, and confounders. Estimates of θ_i and $\boldsymbol{\beta}$ are substituted into the regression model.

Despite the advantages of parametric modeling described earlier, parametric models have some well-known disadvantages. The model is sensitive to differences in the confounder distributions across providers. The model relating the confounders to the outcome needs to be correctly specified, a difficult task if many confounders are included. However, the inclusion of many confounders is required to meet the unconfoundedness assumption. For instance, interaction terms, particularly with the provider indicators, likely add robustness to the model, but with many providers, this may be impossible. Finally, the use of regression modeling alone makes it difficult to assess covariate balance and overlap, both required to infer causality.

Nonparametric or semi-parametric models for risk adjustment have emerged that permit the inclusion of many confounders and relax other assumptions about functional forms. These approaches generally do not produce regression coefficients, complicating interpretation and model transparency, which may be a drawback. Machine learning approaches, algorithms that nonparametrically or semi-parametrically estimate a parameter by *learning* from the data, are attractive options given their flexibility in functional form and less reliance on parametric assumptions. These approaches are briefly described in Section 19.6.

19.5.2 Using the Provider Assignment Mechanism

Rather than modeling the outcome–provider relationship directly, the provider assignment mechanism can be used to balance covariates across providers and assess positivity. Two distinct approaches have been adopted. The first *models* the treatment assignment mechanism to create a balancing score and uses the score to match, weight, or stratify units in the sample. The second approach avoids modeling the treatment assignment mechanism by finding matches or weights that directly optimize prespecified constraints on the empirical distribution of the confounders. The second approach (1) avoids model misspecification problems associated with defining the functional form of the relationship between confounders and treatment assignment, and (2) does not make any distributional assumptions.

Why focus on the treatment assignment mechanism alone? Because the outcome plays no role in the estimation of the assignment mechanism, there is some protection against overfitting. Researchers can work iteratively on estimating q_{ij} to achieve balance across providers while being blinded to the outcomes. Modeling the assignment probability avoids any bias introduced by manipulating the outcome regression model.

A balancing score, b, is a function of the confounders for which, conditional on the value of the score, the probability of receiving care by provider i is independent of the confounders, for example, $H_{ij} \perp \mathbf{X}_{ij} \mid b(\mathbf{X}_{ij})$. This means that within groups of patients having the same value of the balancing score, the distribution of the confounders among the providers is the same. Ideally, the balancing score is of lower dimension than the dimension of $\mathbf{X}_{ij}$. The score is defined as

$$q_{ij}(\mathbf{X}_{ij}) = q(H_{ij} = 1 \mid \mathbf{X}_{ij}) \text{ such that } \sum_{i=1}^{I} q_{ij} = 1. \tag{19.18}$$

The balancing score permits the elimination of the full set of confounders so that conditioning only on a single scalar score is required. The function q characterizes the probability that patient j is treated by provider i. The most familiar balancing score is the *propensity score*, although there are other such scores. Like outcome regression modeling, parametric or nonparametric models or machine learning algorithms may be employed to infer the provider assignment mechanism. A desirable property of the propensity score is that it reduces bias in the estimation of effects for every linear combination of the observed confounders. Importantly, the balancing score provides estimators of causal effects that are simple functions of the balancing scores and the observed outcomes, which may be easier to understand than a parametric regression model.

19.5.2.1 Stratification Using Balancing Scores

Stratification uses balancing scores, $q_{ij}(\mathbf{X}_{ij})$, to divide the sample into S strata such that patients from all providers are balanced to the confounders within each stratum. Within each stratum, an effect is estimated, and then the effect estimates are combined across the strata. Let g_s, $s = 1, 2, \ldots, S$ represent the value of the balancing score defining the stratum, and let $g_0 = 0$ and $g_S = 1$. Within a stratum, suppose there are N_s observations. The average effect of provider i is

$$\delta(s)_{\mathrm{ATE},i} = \frac{\sum_{j:G_{ij}(s)=1} Y_{ij} H_{ij}}{\sum_{j:G_{ij}(s)=1} H_{ij}} - \frac{\sum_{j:G_{ij}(s)=1} Y_{ij}(1 - H_{ij})}{\sum_{j:G_{ij}(s)=1}(1 - H_{ij})}, \tag{19.19}$$

where $G_{ij}(s) = 1$ if $g_{s-1} < q_{ij} < g_s$ and 0 otherwise. The overall ATE for provider i averages the stratum-specific estimates,

$$\hat{\delta}_{\mathrm{ATE},i} = \frac{1}{N} \sum_{s=1}^{S} N_s \delta(s)_{\mathrm{ATE},i}. \tag{19.20}$$

Stratification using balancing scores inherits all the advantages of balancing scores. It may be difficult to find patients from every provider in a stratum once the strata have been defined. This, in itself, provides valuable information about the positivity assumption. When this occurs, then the strata boundaries are changed to include all providers. However, increasing the boundaries may introduce confounder imbalance.

19.5.2.2 Weighting

Under the assumption of unconfoundedness, the potential outcomes for individual j treated by provider i versus not treated by i, are

$$Y_{ij}(H_{ij} = 1) = \frac{Y_{ij} H_{ij}}{q_{ij}(\mathbf{X}_{ij})} \text{ and } Y_{ij}(H_{ij} = 0) = \frac{Y_{ij}(1 - H_{ij})}{1 - q_{ij}(\mathbf{X}_{ij})}; i \neq i*. \quad (19.21)$$

Examination of Eq. 19.21 reveals that the potential outcome for an individual is the observed outcome multiplied by a weight, w_{ij}. Thus, the causal parameter is

$$\frac{\sum_{j=1}^{n_i} H_{ij} Y_{ij} w_{ij}}{\sum_{j=1}^{n_i} H_{ij} w_{ij}} - \frac{\sum_{j=1}^{n_i} (1 - H_{ij}) Y_{ij} w_{ij}}{\sum_{j=1}^{n_i} (1 - H_{ij}) w_{ij}}. \quad (19.22)$$

When estimating the ATE, the weight is

$$w_{ij}^{\text{ATE}} = \frac{H_{ij}}{q_{ij}(\mathbf{X}_{ij})} + \frac{1 - H_{ij}}{1 - q_{ij}(\mathbf{X}_{ij})}, \quad (19.23)$$

and referred to as *inverse probability of treatment weighting*. When treated by provider i, subject j's outcome is weighted by the inverse of the balancing score, whereas if treated by a different provider, the subject's outcome is weighted by the inverse of 1 - balancing score. The construction of the weights depends on the causal parameter. For instance, when assessing the ATT for provider i,

$$w_{ij}^{\text{ATT}} = H_{ij} + \frac{(1 - H_{ij}) q_{ij}(\mathbf{X}_{ij})}{1 - q_{ij}(\mathbf{X}_{ij})}. \quad (19.24)$$

A subject treated by provider i has her outcome weighted by one, whereas if she is treated by a different provider, her outcome is weighted by the odds of treatment by provider i.

The average treatment effect of provider i can be estimated as

$$\delta_{\text{ATE},i} = \frac{1}{N} \left(\sum_{j:H_{ij}=1}^{N} \hat{w}_{ij}^{\text{ATE}} Y_{ij} - \sum_{j:H_{ij}=0}^{N} \hat{w}_{ij}^{\text{ATE}} Y_{ij} \right). \quad (19.25)$$

The estimator in Eq. 19.25 is the Horvitz–Thompson estimator ([48]), although other estimators could be used. Like outcome regression modeling, weights can be sensitive to differences in the confounder distributions across providers that lead to very large or very small weights. The stratification approach minimized this problem through the aggregation of patients into strata. Different approaches have been proposed to address extreme weights. For example, *overlap* weights ([49]) create weights that downweight units in the tails of the propensity score distributions. For the ATE, the overlap weights are $1 - q_{ij}(\mathbf{X}_{ij})$ for those treated by provider i and $q_{ij}(\mathbf{X}_{ij})$ for those not treated at provider i. These weights up-weight units with a high probability of receiving treatment by provider i or not by provider i and down-weight units having probabilities in the tails of the distribution of $q_{ij}(\mathbf{X})$.

19.5.2.3 Matching

Matching is a conceptually simple approach for risk adjustment and enjoys a long history. The interested reader should consult Stuart [50] and references therein for the use of matching in causal inference. A key advantage of matching is the avoidance of extrapolation; inferences are based on observations inside rather than outside of the data. In this way, the unit of analysis remains intact [51]. If for each patient treated by provider i, another patient treated by a provider other than i, having the same values of all the confounders, could be found, confounder balance and overlap are automatically achieved. The problem, of course, is that with many confounders, matching exactly is nearly impossible. Balancing scores thus plays a critical role in matching units. Balancing scores may be based on a model for the treatment assignment mechanism or obtained by solving an optimization problem (see Section 19.6.1).

To create match sets, several decisions must first be made. These include determining the *structure* of the matches: Will the matches be one-to-one (matched pairs) or one-to-many (matched sets)? The algorithm for finding matches needs to be selected, and several algorithms exist, such as *greedy* matching or *optimal* matching. Not all matches may be close enough to be considered good matches. Typically, the closeness of the match is restricted using a propensity caliper or some other distance metric. A value of the distance metric is selected such that units with distances larger than a selected threshold distance will not be considered valid matches (**Box 19.2**). A comparison of observations matched with observations unmatched will be important to understand the generalizability of findings.

Many matching approaches exist and are too numerous to describe. These include *coarsened exact* matching, *genetic* matching, *balance optimization subset selection*, *optimal matching with refined covariate balance*, and *cardinality* matching (see Stuart [50] for a comprehensive assessment of matching approaches).

19.5.3 Combined Approaches

The individual approaches described can be combined to protect against violations of some of the assumptions. For instance, a regression model could be estimated

Box 19.2 Distance measures to define closeness of matches

1. Mahalanobis metric for subject j, provider i

$$d(\mathbf{X}_{ij}, \mathbf{X}_{i*j*}) = (\mathbf{X}_{ij} - \mathbf{X}_{i*,j*})\Sigma^{-1}(\mathbf{X}_{ij} - \mathbf{X}_{i*,j*})^T, \qquad (19.26)$$

where Σ is a $p \times p$ weighted sum of the within-provider i sample covariance matrix of the confounders and the covariance matrix of the confounders of all other providers combined. A match selected if $d(\mathbf{X}_{ij}, \mathbf{X}_{i*j*}) < D$ where D is a threshold.

2. Propensity Caliper is defined as $D* = c \times \sqrt{\mathrm{Var}(\mathrm{logit}(\hat{p}_{ij}))}$ where c is a selected constant. If

$$d(\mathbf{X}_{ij}, \mathbf{X}_{i*j*}) = p_{ij} - p_{i*j*} < D*, \qquad (19.27)$$

the match is selected.

within strata defined by the balancing score if some confounders remain unbalanced in the strata. Regression could be combined with weighting. A particularly important class of methods is *double-robust* methods. These approaches yield unbiased estimates if either the treatment model or the outcome model is correctly specified.

One such estimator is the *augmented inverse probability weighted* estimator, characterized as the sum of the weighted estimator and a weighted average of two regression models. An estimator for the ATE is

$$\frac{1}{N}\sum_{j=1}^{N}\left\{\left(\frac{H_{ij}}{q_{ij}(\mathbf{X}_{ij})}Y_{ij}+\frac{1-H_{ij}}{1-q_{ij}(\mathbf{X}_{ij})}Y_{ij}\right)-\frac{H_{ij}-q_{ij}(\mathbf{X}_{ij})}{q_{ij}(\mathbf{X}_{ij})(1-q_{ij}(\mathbf{X}_{ij}))}\right.$$
$$\left.\times\left((1-q_{ij}(\mathbf{X}_{ij}))m(H_{ij}=1,\mathbf{X}_{ij},\beta_1)+q_{ij}(\mathbf{X}_{ij})m(H_{ij}=0,\mathbf{X}_{ij},\beta_0)\right)\right\}. \quad (19.28)$$

19.6 Additional Robust Approaches

The weighting and matching approaches described earlier were model-based. Parametric models were used to estimate propensity scores that serve as weights or for use in matching. Approaches that work with the confounders *directly* to risk-adjust have also been proposed and more straightforwardly tackle the problem of risk-adjustment. Machine learning algorithms have also emerged that can accommodate more confounders and can be more robust than standard approaches.

19.6.1 Optimization Approaches

More recent work using constrained optimization for creating weights has emerged, and these are discussed more in Chapter 26. In the case of the ATT, the overall goal is to find weights, w_{ij}, so that

$$\frac{1}{n_i}\sum_{H_{ij}=1} f(X_{ij})=\frac{1}{N-n_i}\sum_{H_{ij}\neq 1} w_{ij}f(X_{ij}) \quad (19.29)$$

for bounded functions, f and $N=\sum_i n_i$. The optimization algorithms differ in how they measure the imbalance between provider i and all other hospitals and the penalty imposed on the weights. For instance, the *minimal dispersion approximately balancing weights* specify a set of covariate balance moment requirements and then solve for the weights that minimize the variance of the weights subject to those requirements (**Box 19.3**).

In general, the weights are constrained to be non-negative and sum to one for increased interpretability and to prohibit extrapolating outside of the data. Determining the weights requires work, and there is a robust literature on this topic. The interested reader should consult Ben-Michael et al. [53] and Chattopadhyay et al. [54] about weights in general. See Keele et al. [55] and Han et al. [56] for the use of constrained optimization for profiling specifically.

Box 19.3 Minimal dispersion approximately balancing weights [52]

Select optimal weights by solving an optimization problem subject to user-specified constraints. To create weights to estimate the ATT, the optimization problem is

$$\min_{w} \quad \sum_{j:H_{ij}=0} \psi(w_{ij})$$

$$\text{subject to} \quad \left| \sum_{j:H_{ij}=0} w_{ij} B_k(X_{ij}) - \frac{1}{n_i} \sum_{j:H_{ij}=1} B_k(X_{ij}) \right| \leqslant \lambda_k, \quad k = 1, \ldots, K, \tag{19.30}$$

where $B_k(X_{ij})$ is a function of the covariate X such as a mean or other transformation and λ_k is the size of the difference the user will tolerate.

19.6.1.1 Template Matching

A unique matching problem associated with provider profiling when focusing on the ATE is how to balance so many covariates when there are a large number of providers. One clever solution proposed by Silber et al. [57] is the idea of *template matching*. Rather than matching patients of each provider to every other provider, a sample that is representative of the target population, referred to as the template sample, is selected, and patients treated by each provider are matched to the template (Figure 19.2). In the specific application, these authors created a template of n patients that are common to most hospitals.[5] The template is chosen to be as similar as possible to the composition of the overall population of patients across all hospitals. Within each study hospital of interest, n patients are matched to the n-patient template using cardinality matching. This algorithm finds the largest possible number of patients in each hospital and the template with specified patterns of baseline characteristics that represent a target population for analysis. Given the structure of the matching, hospitals can be directly compared, either overall or for specific types of templates (e.g., procedure–patient combinations).

In a companion paper [58] and subsequent [59] work by the authors, they proposed a matching approach to enable estimation of the ATT by using a template based on its specific mix of patients (the ATT). This "indirect standardization" variant (see Volume 1, Chapter 8, "Risk Modeling and Validation") of template matching constructs the template of n patients from the study hospital's population of patients and identifies matches from other hospitals that have similar case mixes.

19.6.2 Machine Learning

Machine learning, the process of using computational algorithms to learn from data, provides an approach to risk adjustment that has many advantages over traditional risk adjustment approaches. The reasons are several-fold. First, machine learning algorithms permit the inclusion of many more confounders than standard regression approaches, helping to bolster the validity of the *no unmeasured confounders assumption*. Second, many algorithms or *learners* permit nonlinear relationships between the confounders and the outcome without having to a priori

[5] An important consequence of this technique is that case-mix distributions that are uncommon at some hospitals are less likely to be included.

Figure 19.2 Template matching for estimating the ATE across hospitals.

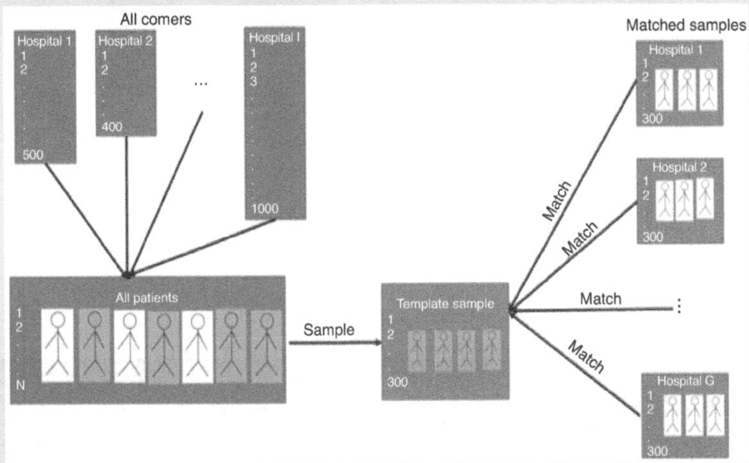

specify the interactions. For instance, *Bayesian Additive Regression Tree* (BART) is a nonparametric Bayesian regression approach that sums over trees where each tree consists of repeated binary splits of confounders—this is discussed in Chapter 26. Third, machine learning can accommodate nonparametric relationships between confounders and outcomes. For instance, *random forests* and *neural networks* assume no parametric relationship between outcomes and confounders. Finally, machine learning algorithms automate cross-validation techniques that mitigate overfitting.

Figure 19.3 contrasts predicted operative mortality probabilities (logit scale) following heart surgery using three different modeling approaches: (1) The *least absolute shrinkage and selection operator* (lasso) is a regression approach selecting the smallest set of covariates that minimizes prediction error subject to a penalty; (2) the BART algorithm that sums predictions from many shallow trees; and (3) a logistic regression model used by the Society for Thoracic Surgeons (STS) for risk adjustment in the study population. Figure 19.3A demonstrates differences in estimated mortality risks for the patients treated in a single hospital. The STS logistic regression model covers a larger range of predictions and places more patients at higher risks than the other two methods. Figure 19.3B–19.3D illustrates between-hospital mortality differences using the same set of four hospitals. Differences in predictions among the four hospitals from the BART approach appear larger than differences using the other approaches.

Additional robustness features can be found in learners that use ensemble methods, e.g., methods that combine predictions from many different learners. For instance, *super learner* [60] averages predictions obtained from several individual learners for each subject. Table 19.2 describes the use of super learner to estimate a binary outcome using five different learners. The weight column indicates how a super learner prediction for a subject is averaged over the five algorithms. Predictions from BART are weighted the highest, and predictions from the lasso

Table 19.2 Example of machine learners and ensemble weights using super learner.

Learner	Weight	Mean cross-validated error
Elastic net	0.25	1.48
Ridge regression	0.15	1.50
BART	0.40	1.46
Lasso regression	0.10	1.51
Gradient boosting	0.10	1.48
Super learner	1.00	1.45

Figure 19.3 Probability of operative mortality using BART, the Lasso, or the STS model based on logistic regression. (A) Compares the expected mortality probabilities (logit scale) for patients treated at a single hospital using 3 different models. (B–D) Display similar distributions for an identical set of four hospitals.

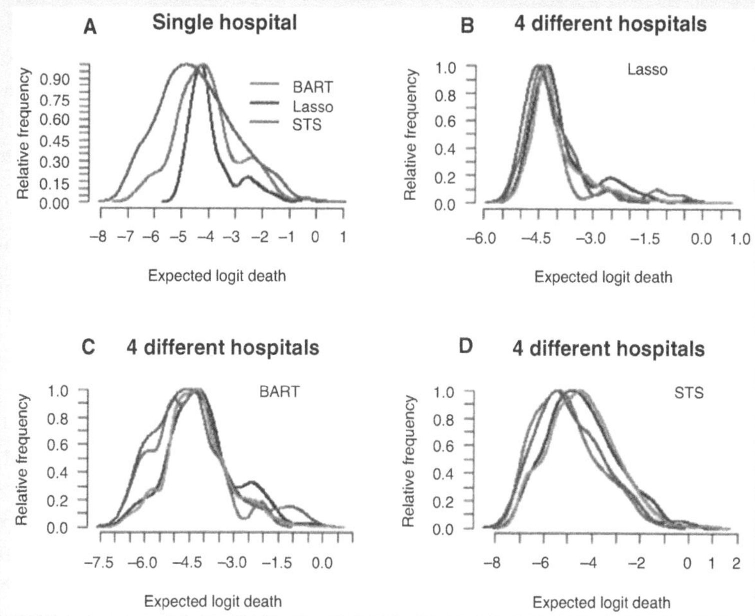

regression and gradient boosting learners are weighted the lowest. The cross-validated error column is a measure of error using the negative log-likelihood when using each algorithm individually and when using the super learner. The error when predicting outcomes using super learner has the smallest error, which is generally always the case. Because machine learning can be used to estimate both the propensity scores, $q_{ij}(\mathbf{X}_{ij})$, and the expected outcomes, $\mathrm{E}(Y_{ij} \mid H_{ij} = 1, \mathbf{X}_{ij})$, their use in causal modeling has increased (see, for instance, Spertus et al. [61]).

19.7 Summary

While the provider profiling problem fits within a causal inference framework, such a framework has not been historically adopted until recently. Moreover, many causal parameters may be of interest. The key assumptions required to draw valid causal inferences include SUTVA assumption, positivity, unconfoundedness, and sample representativeness of the target population. Further discussion of assessment of causal assumptions is provided in Volume 2, Chapter 25, "Model Assessment." There is a large causal inference literature that spans many disciplines. As such, different terminology for the same ideas exists. The SUTVA is sometimes not mentioned, and only the *consistency* assumption is described; the positivity assumption may be described as the *experimental treatment* assignment assumption; and unconfoundedness may be described as *exchangeable* or *ignorable*. When these assumptions are met, the approaches to inference described in this chapter may be used. Machine learning adds a layer of robustness to risk adjustment specifically and to causal modeling in general. The role of nonparametric approaches and Bayesian nonparametric approaches is growing in general, and their potential for profiling is discussed in Chapter 26.

CHAPTER TWENTY

Introduction to Hierarchical Linear Models

The historical evolution of hierarchical models, and their application to provider profiling are described in Volume 1, Chapter 3, "History and Evolution of Healthcare Performance Measurement." This chapter focuses on the key underpinnings of hierarchical models, which involve modeling random and systematic effects at each level of the hierarchy using a probability model. For instance, differences in provider quality may be due to measured and unmeasured confounders, sampling variation, and true differences in quality. Many different statistical approaches have been used to characterize these sources of variation, including dummy variables to represent each hospital or random effects. In this chapter, we outline the structure of hierarchical models, focusing on a linear regression model. Hierarchical models for binary and other non-linear outcomes are discussed in Volume 2, Chapter 21, "Hierarchical Generalized Linear Models." Here, we formalize notation, discuss the assumptions associated with a hierarchical model, and then introduce an example to illustrate ideas. The interpretation of the model parameters is next described, and provider-specific parameters are developed.

20.1 Notation and Structure

Without loss of generality, assume only one level of clustering, e.g., subjects clustered or nested within providers. Let Y_{ij} denote an outcome for the jth subject treated by the ith provider for $i = 1, \ldots, I$ providers, and suppose each provider treats n_i subjects. We let $\mathbf{x}_{ij} = (x_{1ij}, x_{2ij}, \ldots, x_{Pij})$ denote a P-dimensional vector of subject-specific covariates and $\mathbf{w}_i = (w_{1i}, \ldots, w_{Qi})$ denote a Q-dimensional vector of provider characteristics. A hierarchical model is a regression model defined for each level of clustering in the *hierarchy*.

Stage I (patient-level, within-provider model). Assume that

$$Y_{ij} \mid \boldsymbol{\theta}_i, \boldsymbol{\phi}, \mathbf{x}_{ij} \overset{indep.}{\sim} f(Y_{ij} \mid \boldsymbol{\theta}_i, \boldsymbol{\phi}, \mathbf{x}_{ij}), \tag{20.1}$$

where $\boldsymbol{\theta}_i$ is a vector of provider-specific parameters, $\boldsymbol{\phi}$ is a vector of parameters common to all providers, and f represents a distribution. The notation "|" denotes *conditioning*, the distribution of Y assuming we know the values of ($\boldsymbol{\theta}_i$, $\boldsymbol{\phi}$, and $\mathbf{x}_{ij}$).

Stage I reflects the assumption that if we *know* the values of $\boldsymbol{\theta}_i$, $\boldsymbol{\phi}$, and $\mathbf{x}_{ij}$, the outcome for subject j treated by provider i is *independent* of the outcomes of all other subjects treated by the provider. The parameter $\boldsymbol{\theta}_i$ is also denoted as *random effect*. A random effect is a parameter that has a probability distribution and introduces heterogeneity in the outcomes. Thus, *random* refers to variability in the parameter and not to a sampling strategy. Often, $\boldsymbol{\theta}_i$ is a scalar representing a random intercept. However, $\boldsymbol{\theta}_i$ may also represent a vector of regression coefficients associated with patient characteristics. For instance, $\boldsymbol{\theta}_i$ may include a random intercept and a random age coefficient. A random age coefficient implies that the association of age and outcome varies across providers.

Stage II (provider-level, between-provider model). Assume that the vector of provider-specific parameters is related to a vector of provider characteristics. Then

$$\boldsymbol{\theta}_i \mid \boldsymbol{\alpha}, \mathbf{w}_i \overset{indep.}{\sim} g(\boldsymbol{\theta}_i \mid \boldsymbol{\alpha}, \mathbf{w}_i), \tag{20.2}$$

where g is a distribution, $\boldsymbol{\alpha}$ is a vector of *hyperparameters*, and $\boldsymbol{\theta}_i$ is assumed to be independent across i. If no provider-level covariates are included, then $\boldsymbol{\theta}_i \sim g(\theta_i \mid \boldsymbol{\alpha})$ in which case the provider-specific parameters are said to be *completely exchangeable*. Exchangeability implies that a priori, there are no reasons to systematically differentiate among $\boldsymbol{\theta}_1, \boldsymbol{\theta}_2, \ldots, \boldsymbol{\theta}_I$. Thus, a hierarchical model is given by a series of probability statements and assumptions:

$$Y_{ij} \mid \boldsymbol{\theta}_i, \boldsymbol{\phi}, \mathbf{x}_{ij} \overset{indep.}{\sim} f(Y_{ij} \mid \boldsymbol{\theta}_i, \boldsymbol{\phi}, \mathbf{x}_{ij}),$$
$$\boldsymbol{\theta}_i \mid \boldsymbol{\alpha}, \mathbf{w}_i \overset{indep.}{\sim} g(\boldsymbol{\theta}_i \mid \boldsymbol{\alpha}, \mathbf{w}_i).$$

A fully Bayesian specification places prior distributions on the hyperparameters $\boldsymbol{\alpha}$ and on $\boldsymbol{\phi}$. We defer the discussion of the prior distributions for the hyperparameters to Volume 2, Chapter 24, "Inference for Hierarchical Generalized Linear Models."

20.1.1 Cross-Classified Hierarchical Model

Thus far, all lower-level units belong to exactly one higher-level unit, for example, patients undergoing bypass surgery at exactly one hospital. There may be situations where lower-level units do not belong to exactly one higher-level unit. For instance, we may be interested in accounting for the quality of the patient's referring physician in addition to the hospital where the surgery was performed. Each hospital, however, will be associated with many different referring physicians. In this instance, higher-level units can be created by crossing hospitals and physicians. In this way, patients belong to exactly one hospital–physician pair. Let j denote subjects and ik denote the ith hospital and kth referring physician. The model becomes

$$Y_{(ik)j} \mid \boldsymbol{\theta}_{(ik)}, \boldsymbol{\phi}, \mathbf{x}_{(ik)j} \overset{indep.}{\sim} f(Y_{(ik)j} \mid \boldsymbol{\theta}_{(ik)}, \boldsymbol{\phi}, \mathbf{x}_{(ik)j}), \tag{20.3}$$

$$\boldsymbol{\theta}_{(ik)} \mid \boldsymbol{\alpha}, \mathbf{w}_i, \mathbf{w}_k^* \overset{indep.}{\sim} g(\boldsymbol{\theta}_{(ik)} \mid \boldsymbol{\alpha}, \mathbf{w}_i, \mathbf{w}_k^*), \tag{20.4}$$

where $\mathbf{w}_i$ and $\mathbf{w}_k^*$ refer to characteristics of the ith hospital and kth referring physician. The notation (ik) is used to denote that $\boldsymbol{\theta}_{(ik)}$ varies independently across both i and k.

20.2 Assumptions

Because hierarchical models are a series of connected regression models, the usual regression modeling assumptions are required. These include distributional assumptions to specify $f(\cdot)$ and $g(\cdot)$; the functional form of the covariates, $\mathbf{x}_{ij}$ and $\mathbf{w}_i$; additivity of covariates; and various independence assumptions.

The choice of f will be made based on the observed data, and in this chapter, we assume the outcomes are normally distributed. Binary outcomes, such as death, and counts, such as the number of hospital readmissions, arise from distributions other than the normal and are discussed in Volume 2, Chapter 21, "Hierarchical Generalized Linear Models." As in any regression model, the choice and appropriateness of f depend on the data type. The independence assumptions are also important. The Stage I outcomes are assumed to be conditionally independent within each provider, meaning once we know the provider-specific effects, the patient outcomes are independent. When would this assumption not hold? Conditional independence may not hold if there is a surgeon effect in addition to the hospital effect. For instance, we may expect the outcomes of patients treated by the same surgeon within a hospital to be more related than the outcomes of patients treated by two different surgeons within the same hospital.

The distribution of the random effects is particularly important in assessing providers, and the choice of g may not be obvious. The random effects, $\boldsymbol{\theta}_i$, represent *associations* between patient covariates and outcomes; the random intercept is the average value of the outcome when all the covariates are set to 0. It may be reasonable to assume that the distribution of the components of $\boldsymbol{\theta}$ is symmetric, implying some values higher and some values lower than an average. For covariate effects, centering the random effect distribution on 0 implies there is no relationship between the covariate and the outcome, but the associations could also be negative or positive. Candidates for g include the Gaussian distribution or a low-degree-of-freedom t-distribution; completely non-parametric forms of g are also possible. The t-distribution has thicker tails compared to the Gaussian distribution and will accommodate more "outlying" hospital random effects. Mixtures of Gaussian and t-distributions or semi-parametric distributions [62] have also been proposed.

An additional assumption requires that the random effects be uncorrelated with the patient-level covariates [63]. If this assumption is violated, then the estimators for $\boldsymbol{\phi}$ and $\boldsymbol{\theta}_i$ can be biased. Discussion of confounding of cluster effects with within-cluster covariates can be found in several papers, most unrelated to provider profiling [64–68]. Kalbfleisch and Wolfe (2013) [69], a paper that does involve profiling, argued that in hospital performance assessments, the assumption that the random effects are uncorrelated with patient-level covariates could be violated because sicker patients are more likely to be treated at specific hospitals. Berlin et al. [65] suggested reparametrization of the patient-level covariates into a within-hospital component and a between-hospital component through the use of covariate centering to eliminate this dependence.

20.3 Hierarchical Linear Regression

Suppose Y_{ij} is a patient-reported satisfaction score measured at hospital discharge and $\mathbf{x}_{ij}$ includes patient age at hospital admission, sex, and a measure of admission

Figure 20.1 Patient hospital satisfaction scores. Scatterplots of patient scores by age at admission, admission severity, and sex for 1,977 patients treated at 20 hospitals. Barplot provides distribution of the number of patients per hospital.

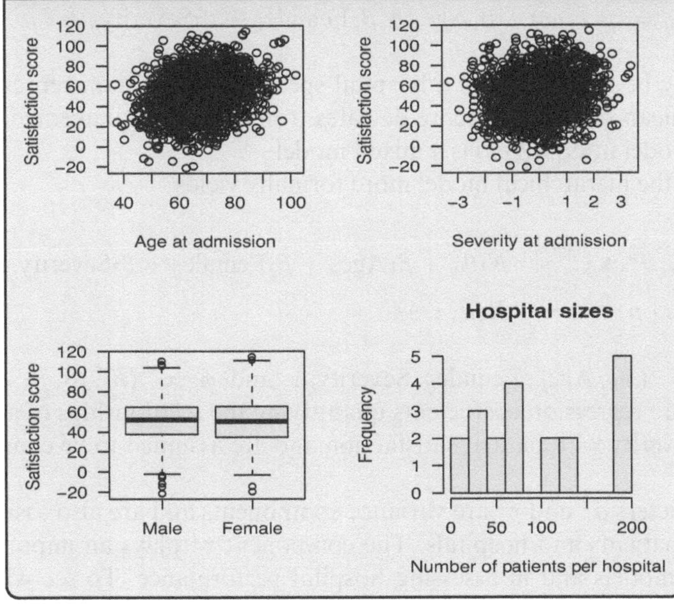

severity. Figure 20.1 provides a summary of data for 1,977 patients treated at 20 hospitals. Higher values of Y_{ij} correspond to higher satisfaction, and higher values of the severity score correspond to sicker patients. The sample consists of 30% women, the mean patient age is 68 years, and patient severity ranges from -3 to 3. The sample mean satisfaction score is 51 (standard deviation = 21). The number of patients per hospital ranges from 12 to 195, with 50% of the hospitals treating fewer than 78 patients. Across hospitals, the mean satisfaction score ranged from 46 to 55.

Assume that

$$Y_{ij} = \theta_{0i} + \beta_1 \text{Age}_{ij} + \beta_2 \text{Female}_{ij} + \beta_3 \text{Severity}_{ij} + \epsilon_{ij},$$

where only the intercept varies across hospitals and ϵ_{ij} reflects patient-specific error unaccounted by the patient covariates. Assume that $\epsilon_{ij} \sim N(0, \sigma^2)$ and is independent across subjects if we knew θ_{0i}. Variation among patients treated within a hospital, σ^2, is assumed constant across hospitals. This implies that after removing the effects of patient covariates, variability across patient satisfaction scores is the same, regardless of where the patient was treated. The f in Eq. (20.1) is a Gaussian density. This type of Stage I model is referred to as a *random intercept* model. A random intercept model assumes that the coefficients of patient-level covariates do not vary across hospitals but that the average (risk-adjusted) hospital score does vary across hospitals. To account for between-hospital variation, suppose we assume

$$\theta_{0i} = \mu + \omega_i.$$

We have not included hospital-specific covariates, and ω_i represents hospital-specific error such that $\omega_i \sim N(0, \tau^2)$. The parameter μ represents the average of the hospital-specific satisfaction scores after adjusting for patient age, sex, and admission severity; τ^2 reflects between-hospital variation in the patient-adjusted satisfaction scores. Substituting the hospital model into the patient model results in

$$Y_{ij} = (\mu + \omega_i) + \beta_1 \text{Age}_{ij} + \beta_2 \text{Female}_{ij} + \beta_3 \text{Severity}_{ij} + \epsilon_{ij}. \tag{20.5}$$

Thus, ω_i may be thought of as a hospital-specific residual term representing how hospital i's mean satisfaction score deviates from the hospital average satisfaction score. The model in Eq. (20.5) is a mixed model.

Rewriting the hierarchical model more formally yields

$$\begin{aligned} Y_{ij} \mid \theta_{0i}, \sigma^2, \mathbf{x}_{ij} &\overset{indep.}{\sim} N(\theta_{0i} + \beta_1 \text{Age}_{ij} + \beta_2 \text{Female}_{ij} + \beta_3 \text{Severity}_{ij}, \sigma^2), \\ \theta_{0i} \mid \mu, \tau^2 &\sim N(\mu, \tau^2), \end{aligned}$$

where $\mathbf{x}_{ij} = (x_{0i}, \text{Age}_{ij}, \text{Female}_{ij}, \text{Severity}_{ij})$, and $\boldsymbol{\phi} = (\beta_1, \beta_2, \beta_3; \sigma^2)$. The $\boldsymbol{\beta}$ parameters are regression coefficients quantifying the relationships of age, sex, and admission severity with patient satisfaction and are assumed to be common across hospitals.

The parameters σ^2 and τ^2 are variance components and are also assumed to not vary across patients and hospitals. The component τ^2 plays an important role in hierarchical models and in assessing hospital performance. To see why, suppose $\tau^2 = 0$. This implies that

$$\begin{aligned} \theta_{01} &= \theta_{02} = \cdots = \theta_{0I} = \mu \\ \text{so that } \mathbb{E}(Y_{ij}) &= \mu + \beta_1 \text{Age}_{ij} + \beta_2 \text{Female}_{ij} + \beta_3 \text{Severity}_{ij}. \end{aligned} \tag{20.6}$$

The notation $\mathbb{E}(Y_{ij})$ refers to the *expectation* of the random variable Y_{ij} and expresses the average value of Y_{ij} obtained by integrating or summing over the distribution of the θ_{0i}. Thus, when $\tau^2 = 0$, there are no differences among the $\theta'_{0i}s$, implying that any of the differences among observed hospital satisfaction scores is entirely due to hospital case-mix and random error. In this setting, data may be safely pooled from all hospitals, ignoring which hospital the patient was treated. Estimates obtained in this manner are referred to as *completely pooled estimates*.

Now suppose τ^2 is very large, which implies hospital-specific random effects differ greatly from each other, suggesting patient case-mix alone does not adequately characterize patient satisfaction at each hospital. This could occur for a variety of reasons, one of which may be due to the underlying (latent) quality of care delivered by the hospital. Completely pooling the satisfaction scores across hospitals would be unwise because any information about the hospital would be lost. If hospital sample sizes were sufficiently large, then one option is to use only the satisfaction scores observed at a hospital, for example, taking the mean of the observed scores over patients within the hospital or estimating a separate linear regression model within each hospital. Estimates obtained this way are referred to as *unpooled estimates*.

Figure 20.2 Mean hospital satisfaction scores. **A**: Hospital mean scores by number of patients per hospital. Solid horizontal lines depict 95% confidence intervals; solid vertical line indicates average satisfaction score across hospitals. Number of patients per hospital has been jittered. **B**: Shrinkage factors. **C**: Observed means versus HLM shrinkage estimates.

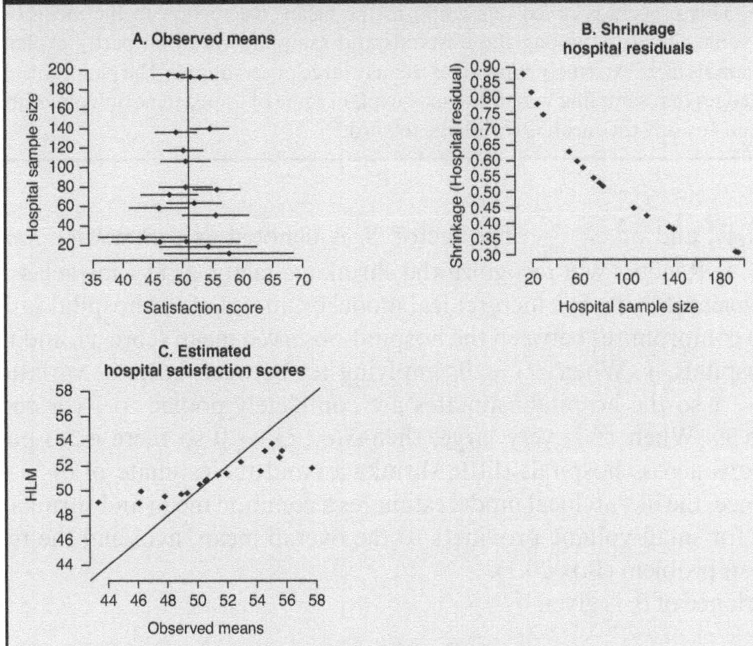

20.3.1 No Adjustment for Patient Risk Factors

Figure 20.2A presents the average observed satisfaction scores, $\bar{y}_i = \frac{1}{n_i}\sum_j y_{ij}$, and corresponding 95% confidence intervals for each hospital. The scores are unadjusted because no accounting for patient-level covariates has been made. Because these estimates use only data observed in the hospital, they are (completely) unpooled estimates. The widths of the confidence intervals vary by hospital sample size: The width for the smallest hospital ($n = 12$) is four times the width of the largest hospital ($n = 195$). The solid vertical line is the average satisfaction score of the 20 hospital-specific means, which is 51. Of course, some hospitals have lower-than-average satisfaction scores while others have higher-than-average satisfaction scores. These results can be obtained using R from fitting a linear model with hosp.id as a factor and removing the intercept term

```
lm(outcome ~ factor(hosp.id) - 1, data=lindata.set)
```

Now consider a hierarchical model. The unadjusted estimated hospital-specific satisfaction score is given by

$$\hat{\theta}_i \mid \bar{y}_i, \tau^2 = \hat{S}(\sigma_i, \tau)\bar{\bar{y}} + (1 - \hat{S}(\sigma_i, \tau))\bar{y}_i \text{ where } \hat{S}(\sigma_i, \tau) = \frac{\hat{\sigma}_i^2}{\hat{\sigma}_i^2 + \hat{\tau}^2}, \tag{20.7}$$

Box 20.1 Regression to the mean

While there is some similarity in outcomes among the hospitals (otherwise, why would we compare them!), we expect to see some differences in the hospital-specific outcomes. In fact, there may be some very large or very small hospital mean outcomes even when all hospitals treat identical patients. A hospital with a very high satisfaction score in one year may have a lower satisfaction score in the following year even if nothing changed between years one and two. This process is called regression to the mean. Regression to the mean occurs if there is some similarity among the hospitals and sampling variation partly explains why some hospitals have extremely small or extremely large observations. The hierarchical model acknowledges that sampling variability may explain some of the extreme outcomes observed. Regression-toward-the-mean is shrinkage toward $\bar{\bar{y}}$.

$\bar{\bar{y}} = \frac{1}{I}\sum_i \bar{y}_i$, and $\sigma_i^2 = \frac{\sigma^2}{n_i}$. The factor S_i is denoted as a *shrinkage factor* with $0 \leqslant S_i \leqslant 1$. Readers will recognize the shrinkage factor as (1 - intraclass correlation coefficient [ICC]). The hierarchical model estimates of the hospital satisfaction scores are compromises between the hospital-observed mean score, $\bar{y}_i$, and the mean across hospitals, $\bar{\bar{y}}$. When $\tau^2 = 0$, implying no between-hospital variation, then $S(\sigma_i, \tau) = 1$ so the hospital estimates are completely pooled to $\bar{\bar{y}}$ (or completely shrunk to $\bar{\bar{y}}$). When τ^2 is very large, then $S(\sigma_i, \tau) = 0$ so there is no pooling of observations across hospitals (little shrinkage) and the estimate of $\hat{\theta}_i = \bar{y}_i$. As a consequence, the hierarchical model estimates a common mean and shrinks hospital estimates for small-volume providers to the overall mean, avoiding the regression to the mean problem (Box 20.1).

The variance of θ_i is given by

$$\sigma_i^2(1 - S(\sigma_i, \tau)). \tag{20.8}$$

Because $0 \leqslant S_i \leqslant 1$, the variance of θ_i will always be smaller than the variance of $\bar{y}_i$. This is a particularly important feature when interest is on the Stage II units, for example, the hospitals.

The R code for estimating the hierarchical model is

```
lmer(outcomes ~ (1 |hosp.id),data=lindata.set)
```

obtained from the package lme4. This function adopts a *mixed model formulation* as presented in Eq. (20.5),

$$Y_{ij} = \mu + \omega_i + \epsilon_{ij},\ \omega_i \sim N(0, \tau^2),\ \text{and}\ \epsilon_{ij} \sim N(0, \sigma^2).$$

The lmer function estimates the parameters using restricted maximum likelihood (discussed in Volume 2, Chapter 24, "Inference for Hierarchical Generalized Linear Models"). The estimate of τ^2 is 4.8 and $\hat{\sigma}^2 = 417$. In the mixed model formulation, the terms ω_i, "hospital residuals," are shrunk to 0 so that

$$\widehat{\omega}_i = \widehat{S}(\sigma_i, \tau) \times 0 + (1 - \widehat{S}(\sigma_i, \tau))(\bar{y}_i - \bar{\bar{y}}). \tag{20.9}$$

The shrinkage factor for each hospital residual is displayed in Figure 20.2B. The mean shrinkage factor is 0.53, ranging from 0.31 to 0.88. The largest value, 0.88, corresponds to the hospital with the smallest sample size ($n = 12$ patients). For this hospital, ω_i is shrunk 88% to 0 from its "observed" deviation from the overall mean. However, even the hospital residual at the largest hospital ($n = 195$) is shrunk by

31% from its residual to 0. Figure 20.2C contrasts the observed means with the estimated means, $\widehat{\mu}+\widehat{\omega}_i$, obtained from the HLM. The distance from the 45-degree line indicates the difference between the two estimates.

20.3.2 Adjustment for Patient Risk Factors

The risk-adjusted hospital-specific satisfaction scores are the terms $\widehat{\beta}_{0i}$ obtained from the linear regression model

$$Y_{ij} = \left(\sum_{i=1}^{H} \beta_{0i} I_{ij}\right) + \beta_1 \text{Age}_{ij} + \beta_2 \text{Female}_{ij} + \beta_3 \text{Severity}_{ij}$$
$$+ \epsilon_{ij};\ \epsilon_{ij} \sim N(0, \sigma^2), \tag{20.10}$$

where $H_{ij} = 1$ if patient j was treated in hospital i and 0 otherwise. This is Eq. (19.17) using the identity link. Because we have excluded the overall intercept term, β_{0i} represents the average hospital satisfaction score after removing the age, sex, and severity effects for hospital i. The estimates, $\hat{\beta}_{0i}$ are obtained in R using

```
lm(outcomes ~ factor(hosp.id) + cage + female + cseverity - 1,
   data=lindata.set)
```

As expected, the hospital-specific satisfaction estimates adjusted for patient characteristics differ from those obtained without adjustment: The average difference between unadjusted and adjusted estimates was -0.59 points (about 0.08 standard deviations). Thus, adjusting for patient factors, on average, decreased the hospital-specific estimates and shortened their confidence intervals. The estimated regression coefficients associated with the patient characteristics are reported in Table 20.1 and indicate that older and sicker patients are more satisfied with the care they receive compared to younger and healthier patients. On average, females are less satisfied by about 1.5 points compared to males. The estimate of $\sigma^2 = (19.53)^2$.

The error term, $\epsilon_{ij} \sim N(0, \sigma^2)$, conveys four important assumptions. First, we assume that the errors are normally distributed. This assumption seems plausible if

Table 20.1 Estimated regression parameters. Higher values of the severity score correspond to higher patient satisfaction. Age and severity are mean-centered. By construction, the linear regression model assumes there is no between-hospital variation.

		Linear regression		Hierarchical regression	
Covariate	**True value**	**Estimate**	**Standard error**	**Estimate**	**Standard error**
Intercept	50	NA	NA	51.5	0.75
Age, years	0.50	0.56	0.05	0.56	0.05
Female	−1.20	−1.51	0.97	−1.40	0.97
Severity	2.50	2.60	0.45	2.59	0.45
Standard deviation					
$\hat{\sigma}$	20	19.53		19.54	
$\hat{\tau}$	4	0		2.15	

we have included the relevant covariates, and let's assume we have done so. Second, the functional form of how the patient covariates are related to patient satisfaction scores is assumed to be additive and linear in the regression coefficients. Hospitals have their own "baseline satisfaction score," which is adjusted up or down in an additive manner by patient characteristics. Third, the variance of the error terms is constant across patients and across hospitals. Perhaps a more plausible assumption for the within-hospital error is to permit it to vary across hospitals, for example, $\sigma^2 = \sigma_i^2$. For instance, assuming $\sigma_i^2 = k_i\sigma^2$ permits a common variance component that varies by a factor specific to each hospital. More complex parameterizations are also possible. For instance, we could model the hospital-specific variance component as a function of hospital characteristics, w_i, or patient characteristics such as $\sigma_i = \exp(\gamma_1 \text{female}_{ij} + \gamma_2 w_i)$. Another assumption made when using the linear regression model is that the satisfaction scores are independent among patients treated within the *same* hospital as well as independent among patients treated at *different* hospitals. Assuming that satisfaction scores from two patients treated at different hospitals are sensible. However, assuming independence between patient satisfaction scores from two patients treated within the same hospital does not seem sensible at all. The conceptual model for assessing the quality of hospital care maintains that patients within a hospital are exposed to that hospital's "quality," so we expect, after adjusting for patient characteristics, patient outcomes to be correlated.

The hierarchical linear regression model is estimated in R using

```
lmer(outcomes ~ (1 |hosp.id) + cage + female + cseverity,
    data=lindata.set)
```

The regression coefficients do not differ meaningfully between the linear regression model and the HLM (Table 20.1), and the within-patient variance is the same. The between-hospital variation is set to 0 in the linear regression model but estimated as $(4.61)^2$ in the HLM. The hospital residuals, $\widehat{\omega}_i$, now involve the covariates, $\bar{\mathbf{x}}_i = \frac{1}{n_i}\sum_{j=1}^{n_i} \mathbf{x}_{ij}$,

$$\widehat{\omega}_i = \widehat{S}(\sigma_i, \tau) \times 0 + (1 - \widehat{S}(\sigma_i, \tau))(\bar{y}_i - \bar{\mathbf{x}}_i\boldsymbol{\beta}). \tag{20.11}$$

20.4 Interpreting the Variance Components

The variance components in the HLM, σ^2 and τ^2, may be used to characterize between-provider variability in a number of different ways.

20.4.1 The ICC

The intraclass correlation coefficient (ICC) is a common measure used to characterize similarity among measurements and is defined as

$$0 \leqslant \frac{\tau^2}{\sigma^2 + \tau^2} = 1 - S(\sigma, \tau) \leqslant 1. \tag{20.12}$$

A small value of the ICC indicates less "similarity" among patients within hospitals (so shrinkage to the overall mean is large), whereas a higher ICC value suggests more within-hospital similarity (less shrinkage to the overall mean). In the latter case, hospital estimates will rely more on their data rather than all data. In our example, the ICC is small, 0.012, and represents the correlation of satisfaction scores between 2 patients treated within the same hospital.

Alternatively, the ICC can be interpreted as the fraction of the total variance *attributed* to the hospital. If all patients from the same hospital reported identical satisfaction scores, then the ICC would be 1. The ICC would be 0 if satisfaction scores from patients treated in the same hospital are no more similar than scores from patients treated at different hospitals. W

20.4.2 The IUR

Examination of Table 20.1 indicates the residual variance at the patient level is $19.5^2 = 382$, which is larger than the hospital-level variance (4.61) suggesting that the hospital effect may be unimportant. Is this a reasonable interpretation? The inter-unit reliability measure compares the "unit" (in this case, the hospital) variance to measurement error. The measurement error is calculated as the residual variance divided by the average hospital sample size, $\bar{n}$,

$$\frac{\tau^2}{\tau^2 + \frac{\sigma^2}{\bar{n}}}. \qquad (20.13)$$

The difference between the ICC (Eq. 20.12) and the inter-unit reliability (IUR) (Eq. 20.13) is that the IUR is focused on characterizing how well we can distinguish the outcomes of one hospital from the outcomes of another hospital. An $IUR = 0$ implies that all the variability in the hospital measure is due to measurement error, whereas if $IUR = 1$, then all the variability is due to real differences in hospital outcomes. A suggested rule of thumb argues that IUR values of 70% or higher at the cluster level (vs. individual level) are sufficiently reliable [70]. In our example, the average number of patients per hospital is 99, and the patient-level variance is 382, so the variance of the satisfaction scores for a hospital of average sample size is 3.56. The inter-hospital reliability is $0.54 = 4.61/(4.61 + 3.56)$, suggesting that the satisfaction scores may not adequately distinguish patient satisfaction of one hospital from another.

Some authors have criticized the IUR [71], arguing large values may mean more patient risk-adjustment is required and small values do not necessarily rule out the measure as useful for profiling. These authors define profiling inter-unit reliability (PIUR) of a measure as the extent to which the measure identifies the same providers as "outliers" when the data are replicated.

20.4.3 Range in Variation

Rather than focusing on variance components alone, a description in the "range" of hospital estimates ([72]; page 168) may be more meaningful. The standard deviation of θ_is from the Stage II Equation, τ, and characterizes the entire distribution of the provider random effects. Recalling that $\theta_i \sim N(0, \tau^2)$, then 95% of the θ_is will lie in the range of $\mu \pm 1.96\tau$ so that the distance between the 97.5% and 2.5% values is $2 \times 1.96 \times \tau$. Using the hierarchical regression output, after adjusting for patient characteristics, compared to patients treated at a low-satisfaction hospital, on average, patients treated at a high-satisfaction hospital are 8.41 points more satisfied with the treatment they received. Given the standard deviation of the patient satisfaction scores is 21, an 8.41-point difference represents an "effect size" of $0.40 = 8.41/21$. Whether an 8.41-point between-hospital difference in satisfaction scores is meaningful is a clinical rather than a statistical decision.

20.4.4 Information Content

Gelman and Hill [26] (page 258) proposed the ratio $\tau^2/\sigma^2 = \gamma$ as a measure of the information content. The ratio represents the strength of the hospital signal relative to sampling error and may be used to characterize the information content given a hospital's sample size. The standard deviation of average outcomes between hospitals, τ, is about the same as the standard deviation of $1/\gamma$ outcomes within a hospital. Roughly, this ratio may be used to determine if the between-hospital model provides more information for hospitals with fewer than $1/\gamma$ patients. In our example, $\hat{\gamma}$ is $\frac{2.15^2}{19.54^2} = 0.012$, so that the hospital-specific estimates for hospitals with fewer than $83 = \frac{1}{0.012}$ patients rely more on the overall mean than on their hospital-specific estimates compared to hospitals with more than 83 patients. In our example, 55% of the hospitals treated fewer than 83 patients.

20.4.5 Some Remarks

The calculations of the ICC, IUR, and the signal-to-noise ratio assumed that the within-hospital variance and the number of patients per hospital are the same across hospitals. These assumptions, of course, are typically untrue. Nonetheless, these metrics provide some guidance about differences between hospital outcomes (Table 20.2). Should the patient satisfaction scores be used to compare hospitals, assuming all relevant confounders have been taken into account? Based on the data, only a small percentage (1.2%) of the total variation can be attributed to the hospital, although the inter-hospital reliability is 54%. The range in the hospital-specific estimates is 8.41 points, which may or may not be clinically meaningful. Finally, the hospital satisfaction estimates for about half the hospitals rely more on the average satisfaction score across all hospitals than on their estimates.

Table 20.2 Hospital metrics for patient satisfaction scores.

Metric	Value
Intraclass correlation coefficient	0.012
Inter-unit reliability	0.54
Range	8.41
Information content	83

Range = approximate width of a 95% confidence interval for hospital-specific satisfaction scores; information = hospital sample size threshold below which there is more shrinkage to the overall mean.

20.5 Provider-Specific Parameters

The primary goal in provider profiling is to determine how well a provider is delivering care. Volume 2, Chapter 19, "A Causal Inference Framework," indicated that to answer such questions, a counterfactual outcome is required. Suppose interest is in estimating how well a hospital fared with the patients it treated, that is, the ATT. The expected outcome, ν_i, for the ith provider, is defined conditionally on the provider's random effects and its case-mix. Noting that

$$\nu_i = \underbrace{\frac{1}{n_i}\sum_{j=1}^{n_i} E(Y_{ij} \mid \mathbf{x}_{ij}, \boldsymbol{\theta}_i, \phi)}_{\text{Regression}} \text{ and } \nu_i^C = \underbrace{\frac{1}{n_i}\sum_{j=1}^{n_i} \int_{\boldsymbol{\theta}_i} E(Y_{ij} \mid \mathbf{x}_{ij}, \boldsymbol{\theta}_i, \phi, \boldsymbol{\alpha}) d\boldsymbol{\theta}_i}_{\text{Counterfactual}}, \quad (20.14)$$

the expected outcomes at provider i are the conditional estimate, and the counterfactual outcomes are obtained by averaging the expected outcomes over the random effects of all hospitals, for example, the marginal distribution of Y_{ij}. Returning to the HLM,

$$\begin{aligned} Y_{ij} \mid \theta_{0i}, \sigma^2, \mathbf{x}_{ij} &\overset{indep.}{\sim} N(\theta_{0i} + \beta_1 \text{Age}_{ij} + \beta_2 \text{Female}_{ij} + \beta_3 \text{Severity}_{ij}, \sigma^2), \\ \theta_{0i} \mid \mu, \tau^2, \sigma^2 &\sim N(\mu, \tau^2), \end{aligned}$$

we have

$$\begin{aligned} \nu_i &= \frac{1}{n_i}\sum_{j=1}^{n_i} \mathbb{E}(Y_{ij} \mid \theta_{0i}) = \frac{1}{n_i}\sum_{j=1}^{n_i} (\theta_{0i} + \beta_1 \text{Age}_{ij} + \beta_2 \text{Female}_{ij} + \beta_3 \text{Severity}_{ij}) \text{ and} \\ \nu_i^C &= \frac{1}{n_i}\sum_{j=1}^{n_i} \int_{\boldsymbol{\theta}_i} \mathbb{E}(Y_{ij} \mid \mu) d\boldsymbol{\theta}_i = \frac{1}{n_i}\sum_{j=1}^{n_i} (\mu + \beta_1 \text{Age}_{ij} + \beta_2 \text{Female}_{ij} + \beta_3 \text{Severity}_{ij}). \end{aligned}$$

Thus, Hospital i's quality may be inferred by determining whether $\delta_i = \nu_i - \nu_i^C$ is meaningfully different from zero or if $\frac{\nu_i}{\nu_i^C}$ is meaningfully different from 1. In the HLM,

$$\delta_i = \nu_i - \nu_i^C = \theta_{0i} - \mu,$$

so very large or very small values of δ_i suggest provider i is far from the average. Similarly, in the mixed model formulation of the HLM,

$$\delta_i = \omega_i,$$

so values far from 0 suggest an unusual provider.[1] Figure 20.3 displays a density estimate of the $\widehat{\omega}_i$s using the model that adjusted for age, sex, and severity.

How far is too far? The estimated hospital residuals range from −2.38 to 2.65.[2] We could determine the probability that a provider has unusually low or unusually high outcomes using

[1] If using a linear model (Eq. 20.10) rather than an HLM, researchers have focused on estimating or testing the β_{0i}s. However, because observations are clustered within the provider, ω_i (or conversely $\theta_{0i} - \mu$) is a more sensible parameter given this parameter aligns with the hypothesized data-generating process.

[2] The uncertainty associated with each ω_i has been ignored.

Figure 20.3 Density estimate of hospital residuals. Density estimate of $\widehat{\omega}_i$, $i = 1, 2 \ldots 20$ obtained from the HLM adjusting for age, sex, and severity using the function lmer.

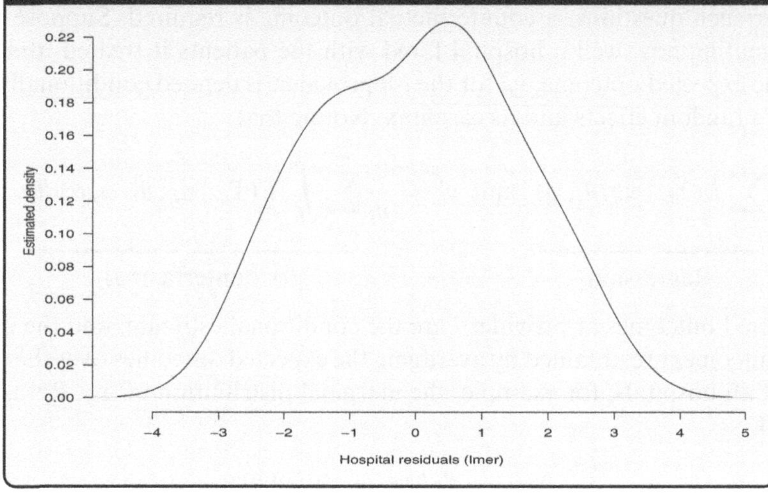

$$\mathbb{P}(\theta_{0i} - \mu > M) \tag{20.15}$$

where M is selected a priori. M could be a percentile of the estimated distribution of $\{\theta_{0i} - \mu; i = 1, 2, \ldots, I\}$ or an absolute difference on the outcome scale. Fully Bayesian approaches are best suited for these calculations, as these approaches can account for the various sources of uncertainty in the estimates, and the calculation of posterior distributions of functions of the parameters is straightforward. Volume 2, Chapter 24, "Inference for Hierarchical Generalized Linear Models," presents posterior summaries for these quantities.

20.6 More than One Random Effect

Our initial model for the patient satisfaction scores assumed one random hospital effect

$$\begin{aligned} Y_{ij} &= \theta_{0i} + \beta_1 \text{Age}_{ij} + \beta_2 \text{Female}_{ij} + \beta_3 \text{Severity}_{ij} + \epsilon_{ij}, \\ \theta_{0i} &= \mu + \omega_i. \end{aligned}$$

Perhaps other hospital random effects exist. For instance, we may hypothesize that some hospitals are better able to handle very complex cases than other hospitals. To reflect this assumption in a model, we permit the relationship between severity at hospital entry and patient satisfaction at discharge to vary across hospitals,

$$Y_{ij} = \theta_{0i} + \beta_1 \text{Age}_{ij} + \beta_2 \text{Female}_{ij} + \theta_{3i} \text{Severity}_{ij} + \epsilon_{ij}, \tag{20.16}$$

$$\theta_{0i} = \mu_0 + \omega_{0i} \text{ and } \theta_{3i} = \mu_3 + \omega_{3i}. \tag{20.17}$$

Now there are two hospital random effects. The interpretation of θ_{0i} remains the same as in the earlier model, that is, the average hospital-specific satisfaction score for a male patient of average age and severity. The parameter θ_{3i} represents the change in the satisfaction score for patients treated at hospital i when increasing patient admission severity by one point. Substituting Eq. (20.17) into Eq. (20.16) yields

$$Y_{ij} = \mu_0 + \beta_1 \text{Age}_{ij} + \beta_2 \text{Female}_{ij} + \mu_3 \text{Severity}_{ij} + (\epsilon_{ij} + \omega_{0i} + \omega_{3i}\text{Severity}_{ij}).$$

Note that the satisfaction error for a patient now varies with the patient's admission severity. We assume $\epsilon_{ij} \sim N(0, \sigma^2)$ and $\omega_{0i} \sim N(0, \tau_0^2)$. With the additional random effect, more assumptions are required for the variance of ω_{3i} and the relationship between ω_{0i} and ω_{3i}. We assume that $\omega_{3i} \sim N(0, \tau_3^2)$ and permit a correlation between ω_{0i} and ω_{3i}

$$\begin{pmatrix} \omega_{0i} \\ \omega_{3i} \end{pmatrix} \sim N\left(\begin{pmatrix} 0 \\ 0 \end{pmatrix}, \begin{pmatrix} \tau_0^2 & \rho\tau_0\tau_3 \\ \rho\tau_0\tau_3 & \tau_3^2 \end{pmatrix}\right). \tag{20.18}$$

The term ρ is a between-hospital correlation parameter. Thus, four "covariance" parameters must be estimated in addition to the regression coefficients: σ which is the unexplained within-hospital standard deviation of the satisfaction scores, τ_0 which is the standard deviation of the hospital intercepts, τ_3 which is the standard deviation of the hospital-specific severity effects, and ρ which is the correlation between the hospital intercepts and hospital severity effects.

20.6.1 Provider-Specific Parameters

With more than one provider random effect, how can quality for a specific provider be defined? Given the multivariate nature of the parameters, it may be worthwhile to determine how far a provider is from other providers. Mahalanobis squared distance, defined as

$$d_i^2 = (\boldsymbol{\theta}_i - \bar{\boldsymbol{\theta}})^\top \Sigma_\theta (\boldsymbol{\theta}_i - \bar{\boldsymbol{\theta}}) \tag{20.19}$$

with $\bar{\boldsymbol{\theta}} = \frac{1}{I}\sum_i (\theta_{0i}, \theta_{3i})^\top$ and $\Sigma_\theta = \frac{1}{I-1}(\boldsymbol{\theta}_i - \bar{\boldsymbol{\theta}})(\boldsymbol{\theta}_i - \bar{\boldsymbol{\theta}})^\top$ is one measure of distance in multivariate space. Large values suggest provider i is "far" from the average across all providers. Similar to the univariate setting, the probability that a provider is far from other providers could be defined as

$$\pi_i = \mathbb{P}(d_i^2 > \xi_{0.95}),$$

where $\xi_{0.95}$ is the 95th percentile of d_i.[3]

20.7 More than Two Levels

The extension to more levels in the hierarchy is straightforward. Suppose we are interested in assessing geographic variation in addition to hospital variation. Let j denote patient, i denote hospital, and k state. In this example, patients are completely nested in the hospital, and hospitals are completely nested within a state. One possible model is

[3] Because a provider has a high π_i does not mean the provider is an outlier. Only by examining the actual values of $\boldsymbol{\theta}_i$ will such a determination be made.

Box 20.2 Cross-classified hierarchical model

Cross-classification of higher level two units, i and k, yields the following random intercept only model

$$\begin{aligned} Y_{(ik)j} &= \theta_{(ik)} + \boldsymbol{\beta}^{\top}\mathbf{x}_{(ik)j} + \epsilon_{(ik)j}, \\ \theta_{(ik)} &= \gamma + \boldsymbol{\alpha}^{\top}\mathbf{w}_i + \boldsymbol{\delta}^{\top}\mathbf{w}_k^* + \omega_i + \zeta_k, \end{aligned}$$

where the error terms are independent.

$$\begin{aligned} Y_{ikj} &= \theta_{ik} + \boldsymbol{\beta}^{\top}\mathbf{x}_{ikj} + \epsilon_{ikj}, \\ \theta_{ik} &= \mu_k + \boldsymbol{\alpha}^{\top}\mathbf{w}_{ik} + \omega_{ik}, \\ \mu_k &= \gamma + \boldsymbol{\delta}^{\top}\mathbf{w}_k^* + \zeta_k. \end{aligned}$$

Assuming conditional independence at each stage and $\epsilon_{ikj} \sim N(0, \sigma_\epsilon^2)$, $\omega_{ik} \sim N(0, \sigma_\omega^2)$, and $\zeta_k \sim N(0, \sigma_\zeta^2)$, then between-hospital variation within state is quantified by σ_ω^2 and between-state variation is σ_ζ^2. The total variance at the hospital level is $\sigma_\omega^2 + \sigma_\zeta^2$, implying the variance due to hospital is $\sigma_\omega^2/(\sigma_\omega^2 + \sigma_\zeta^2)$.

Cross-classification of higher-level units is also possible (Box 20.2).

Coefficients in addition to the intercepts may vary, becoming more computationally complex due to the increased number of variance components and multivariate distributions, but remain conceptually simple.

20.8 Summary

The hierarchical linear model is a natural extension of the linear model and has been represented many different ways for users; see Gelman and Hill (2007) [26] for examples. Such models arise when data are thought to arise from "repeated execution of the same type of random experiment" [73]. While the use of hierarchical linear models in assessing medical providers has been infrequent, mainly because most health outcomes collected are discrete, they are numerous in other fields. The 1982 paper by Laird and Ware [74] introduced random effects model for longitudinal data, treating subjects as clusters (level II) with measurement occasions (level I) nested within subjects. This work demonstrated how the hierarchical model provided a unified approach for modeling clustered data that permitted more flexibility than many of the other approaches used at that time. Meta-analysis, combining information from multiple studies, utilizes hierarchical linear models to pool information to obtain an overall estimate of treatment effects and of estimates from specific studies [75–77]. An interesting use of hierarchical models was described by Dumouchel and Harris [78] for characterizing dose–response functions of lung cancer in humans using experiments in multiple species, humans, and animals, and from multiple types of environmental emissions.

CHAPTER TWENTY-ONE

Hierarchical Generalized Linear Models

Volume 2, Chapter 20, "Introduction to Hierarchical Linear Models," described the hierarchical linear model as an extension of the linear regression model. Linear regression models belong to a larger class of models denoted *generalized linear models* (GLM) that contain regression models for a broad array of outcome distributions, including the normal, binomial, and Poisson. In this chapter, we introduce the *hierarchical generalized linear model* (HGLM) as a natural extension to the hierarchical linear model. We begin with formal statistical representations of GLMs and their connection to HGLMs using a generalized linear mixed modeling (GLLM) framework. This framework for the HGLM is from a frequentist perspective, where regression parameters are fixed unknown quantities. We then present the HGLM in a more general format and introduce the Bayesian framework for HGLMs, where parameters are unknown random quantities. We describe provider-specific parameters for profiling.

21.1 The GLM

A GLM is broadly defined by three components: the *probability* component that specifies the distribution of the outcome, Y, conditional on covariates, $\mathbf{X}$; the *systematic* component, a linear predictor, defined by the linear function of the covariates; and a *link* function that connects the probability component to the systematic component. Letting $\mu = \mathbb{E}(Y \mid X)$, a GLM is given by

1. $Y \mid X_1, X_2, \ldots, X_p \sim f$, where f is from an exponential family,
2. $\eta = \sum_k \beta_k X_k$ (linear predictor), and
3. $\eta = l(\mu)$, where $l(\mu)$ is a monotonic differentiable function referred to as a *link function*.

The probability component of a GLM is assumed to arise from a one-parameter exponential family.[1] Assuming n independent observations, the log-likelihood takes the form

[1] A Bayesian treatment of the GLM is provided at the end of this chapter.

Table 21.1 Link functions for common distributions. n is the denominator.

Distribution	θ	v	Link function	ϕ
Normal, $N(\mu, \sigma^2)$	μ	1	identity	σ^2
Binomial, $Bin(n, \mu)$	$\log(\frac{\mu}{n-\mu})$	$\frac{\mu(n-\mu)}{n}$	logit	$\frac{1}{n}$
Poisson, $Poi(\mu)$	$\log(\mu)$	μ	log	1

$$\sum_{j=1}^{n} \left\{ \frac{y_j\theta - b(\theta) + c(y_j, \phi)}{\phi} \right\}, \tag{21.1}$$

where θ is the *canonical* parameter and is some function of μ, and ϕ is the *dispersion* or scale parameter. Note that

$$\int_y \exp\left\{ \frac{(y\theta - b(\theta)) + c(y, \phi)}{\phi} \right\} dy = 1 \text{ so that } \exp\left\{ \frac{b(\theta)}{\phi} \right\} = \int_y \exp\left\{ \frac{y\theta + c(y, \phi)}{\phi} \right\} dy\,.$$

If ϕ is unknown, y may or may not be from an exponential family. For one parameter exponential models, the mean and variance are

$$\mu = \mathbb{E}(y) = \frac{\partial b(\theta)}{d\theta} \text{ and } v = \text{var}(y) = \phi \frac{\partial^2 b(\theta)}{d\theta^2} = \phi \text{Var}(\mu).$$

Table 21.1 provides common examples of exponential families and their corresponding link functions. The logit link function ensures that variables for which $0 < \mu < 1$ map to the whole real line, while the log link ensures $\mu > 0$.

21.1.1 Example: Normal Model Formulation

If $y_j \sim N(\mu, \sigma^2)$, then

$$\begin{aligned} p(y_j \mid \mu, \sigma^2) &= \frac{1}{\sqrt{2\pi\sigma^2}} \exp\left\{ -\frac{(y_j - \mu)^2}{2\sigma^2} \right\} \\ &= \exp\left\{ \frac{(y_j\mu - \frac{\mu^2}{2})}{\sigma^2} - \frac{1}{2}\left(\frac{y_j^2}{\sigma^2} + \log(2\pi\sigma^2) \right) \right\}. \end{aligned}$$

Referring to Eq. (21.1),

$$\theta = \mu, \;\; \phi = \sigma^2, \;\; b(\theta) = \frac{\theta^2}{2}, \text{ and } c(y, \phi) = -\frac{1}{2}\left[\frac{y_j^2}{\sigma^2} + \log(2\pi\sigma^2) \right].$$

If we have a normal linear regression model, $\theta = \mathbf{x}\boldsymbol{\beta}$.

21.1.2 Example: Binomial Model Formulation

Suppose $y_j \sim$ binomial(n, p) so that

$$\begin{aligned}
p(y_j \mid n, p) &= \binom{n}{y_j} p^{y_j}(1-p)^{n-y_j} \\
&= \exp\left\{ y_j \log(p) + (n-y_j)\log(1-p) + \log\binom{n}{y_j} \right\} \\
&= \exp\left\{ y_j \log\left(\frac{p}{1-p}\right) - n\log\left(\frac{1}{1-p}\right) + \log\binom{n}{y_j} \right\} \\
&= \exp\left\{ n\left[\frac{y_j}{n}\log\left(\frac{p}{1-p}\right) - \log\left(\frac{1}{1-p}\right)\right] + \log\binom{n}{y_j} \right\}.
\end{aligned}$$

Thus, $\theta = \log\left(\frac{p}{1-p}\right)$, $\phi = \frac{1}{n}$, $c(y, \phi) = \log\binom{n}{y_j}$, and

$$\begin{aligned}
b(\theta) = \log\left(\frac{1}{1-p}\right) &= -\log(1-p) = -\log\left(1 - \frac{e^\theta}{1+e^\theta}\right) \\
&= -\log\left(\frac{1}{1+e^\theta}\right) = \log(1+e^\theta).
\end{aligned}$$

For a binomial regression model, $\theta = \mathbf{x}\boldsymbol{\beta}$ and $b(\theta) = \log(1 + \exp(\mathbf{x}\boldsymbol{\beta}))$.

21.2 The HGLM

In a GLMM framework,

$$l(\mu_{ij}) = \beta_{0i} + \sum_{p=1}^{P} \mathbf{x}_{pij}\beta_p \ \text{ where } \ \beta_{0i} \sim N(\mu, \tau^2)$$

is re-expressed as

$$l(\mu_{ij}) = \beta_0 + \sum_{p=1}^{P} \mathbf{x}_{pij}\beta_p + r_i \ \text{ where } \ r_i \sim N(0, \tau^2) \qquad (21.2)$$

where $\beta_0 = \mu$. Eq. (21.2) is a mixed model representation of the hierarchical generalized linear model. For each cluster i, the GLMM models its deviation from the overall mean, β_0. In general, the form of the linear predictor in the GLMM is presented as two components separated into the regression coefficients that are constant across clusters and the regression coefficients that vary across clusters

$$l(\mu_{ij}) = \sum_{p=1}^{P} \mathbf{x}_{pij}\beta_p + \sum_{q=1}^{Q} z_{qij}v(r_i) \ \text{ with } \ \mathbf{z}_{ij} \in \mathbf{x}_{ij}.$$

Note that provider-level covariates, $\mathbf{w}_i$, are included in $\mathbf{x}_{ij}$. In the mixed model setting, $v_i = v(r_i)$ is a monotone function of r_i.

21.2.1 Frequentist Formulation

Lee and Nelder [79] defined the HGLM using a GLMM framework as:

1. Stage I. Conditional on the random effects, r_i, the outcomes are independent and arise from a GLM where $\mathbb{E}(y_{ij} \mid r_i) = \mu_{ij}$, $\text{Var}(y_{ij} \mid r_i) = \phi V(\mu_{ij})$, $\eta_{ij} = l(\mu_{ij}) = \sum_k (\beta_k x_{kij} + z_{kij} v_i)$, and $v_i = v(r_i)$. The log-likelihood is proportional to

$$\sum_{i=1}^{I} \sum_{j=1}^{n_i} \left\{ \frac{y_{ij}\theta_{ij} - b(\theta_{ij}) + c(y_{ij}, \phi)}{\phi} \right\} \tag{21.3}$$

   with $\theta_{ij} = \theta(\mu_{ij})$ and ϕ is a dispersion parameter.
2. Stage II. The random effects are independent and identically distributed from a one-parameter exponential distribution proportional to

$$\sum_{i=1}^{I} \frac{\theta_R(r_i)\psi_R - b_R(\theta_R(r_i))}{\lambda} \tag{21.4}$$

   where, for conjugate distributions,[2] $\mathbb{E}(r_i) = \psi_R$, $\text{Var}(r_i) = \rho \text{V}(\psi_R)$, λ is a dispersion parameter, and where $\theta_R()$ and $b_R()$ are functions.

Several remarks are in order. First, selecting $\theta_R(r_i) = \theta(r_i)$ and $b_R(\theta_R) = b(\theta)$ leads to a *conjugate log-likelihood* for the random effects. A conjugate log-likelihood is not necessary, although having such a log-likelihood permits the use of the joint likelihood of the parameters for estimation (see Volume 2, Chapter 24, "Inference for Hierarchical Generalized Linear Models"). Second, Stage II need not arise from a one-parameter exponential distribution. Volume 2, Chapter 24 discusses the form of Stage II and constraints associated with different inferential approaches.[3] The inferential approach used in this formulation of the HGLM is based on an *extended likelihood.*

21.2.1.1 Example: Normal Stage I and Normal Stage II Model

Assuming $Y_{ij} \mid r_i \sim N(\mu_{ij}, 1)$ with $\mu_{ij} = \mathbf{x}_{ij}\boldsymbol{\beta} + r_i$, the contribution to the log-likelihood for Stage I is

$$\log(f(y_{ij})) \propto \sum_j \left\{ \left(y_{ij}\mu_{ij} - \frac{\mu_{ij}^2}{2} \right) - \frac{1}{2}\left(y_{ij}^2 + \log(2\pi) \right) \right\},$$

so that $\theta_{ij} = \mu_{ij} = \mathbf{x}_{ij}\boldsymbol{\beta} + r_i$, $\phi = 1$, $b(\theta) = \frac{\theta_{ij}^2}{2}$, and $v_i = r_i$. In Stage II, let $r_i \sim N(0, \tau^2)$, then the log-likelihood for Stage II is

$$\log(g(r_i)) \propto \sum_i \frac{r_i^2}{2\tau^2},$$

[2] A conjugate Stage II distribution is such that the density when combined with Stage I, belongs to the same family as the Stage II distribution.

[3] In Bayesian approaches, there are no constraints; rather prior distributions are specified. The Stage II distribution could also include covariates, and hence the identically distributed assumption is also not required.

implying λ in Eq. (21.4) is τ^2. Note that the normal log-likelihood for the random effects is conjugate.

21.2.1.2 Example: Binomial Stage I and Beta Stage II Model

Assume $y_{ij} \mid r_i \sim \text{Bernoulli}(p_{ij})$ so that $\mu_{ij} = p_{ij} = \mathbb{E}(y_{ij} \mid r_i)$ where

$$\log\left(\frac{p_{ij}}{1-p_{ij}}\right) = x_{ij}\beta + v_i \text{ with } v_i = \log\left(\frac{r_i}{1-r_i}\right).$$

The contribution to the log-likelihood for Stage I is

$$\log(f(y_{ij})) \propto \sum_{j=1}^{n_i} y_{ij}(x_{ij}\beta + v_i) - \log\left(1 + \exp(x_{ij}\beta + v_i)\right),$$

so that in Eq. (21.3) $\phi = 1$, $\theta_{ij} = \log\left(\frac{p_{ij}}{1-p_{ij}}\right) = x_{ij}\beta + v_i$, and $b(\theta_{ij}) = \log(1 + \exp(x_{ij}\beta + v_i))$. Assume $r_i \sim \text{Beta}(\alpha, \beta)$ so it has density

$$g(r_i) = \frac{1}{B(\alpha,\beta)} r_i^{\alpha-1}(1-r_i)^{\beta-1} \;\; \alpha > 0, \beta > 0,$$

where $B(\alpha, \beta)$ is the beta function. For the Beta distribution, $\mathbb{E}(r_i) = \psi_R = \frac{\alpha}{\alpha+\beta}$ and $\text{Var}(r_i) = \frac{\psi_R(1-\psi_R)}{1+\alpha+\beta}$. The log-likelihood for Stage II is

$$\begin{aligned}\log(g(r_i)) &\propto \sum_{i=1}^{n_i}\left(\frac{\frac{\alpha}{\alpha+\beta}\log\left(\frac{r_i}{1-r_i}\right) - \log\left(\frac{1}{1-r_i}\right)}{\lambda} - \log(B(\alpha,\beta))\right)\\ &= \sum_{i=1}^{n_i}\left(\frac{\frac{\alpha}{\alpha+\beta}v_i - \log\left(\frac{1}{1-r_i}\right)}{\lambda} - \log(B(\alpha,\beta))\right),\end{aligned}$$

so referring to Eq. (21.4), $\lambda = \frac{1}{\alpha+\beta}$, $\theta_R = \log\left(\frac{r_i}{1-r_i}\right) = v_i$, and $b_R = \log(1 + \exp v_i)$ so that the Beta distribution yields a conjugate log-likelihood.

21.2.1.3 Example: Poisson Stage I and Gamma Stage II Model

Suppose $y_{ij} \mid r_i \sim Pois(\mu_{ij})$, where $\mu_{ij} = \mathbb{E}(y_{ij} \mid r_i) = \text{Var}(y_{ij} \mid r_i)$. Then, the Stage I contribution to the log-likelihood is

$$\log(f(y_{ij})) \propto \sum_{j=1}^{n_i}\left(y_{ij}\log\mu_{ij} - \mu_{ij}\right) \;\text{ where }\; \log\mu_{ij} = x_{ij}\beta + v_i \;\text{ and }\; v_i = \log r_i.$$

Comparing to Eq. (21.3) $\phi = 1$, $\theta_{ij} = \log\mu_{ij}$, and $b(\theta_{ij}) = \exp\theta_{ij}$. A gamma distribution for r_i is conjugate for $y_{ij} \mid r_i$, having density

$$g(r_i) = \left(\frac{1}{\gamma}\right)^{\frac{1}{\gamma}} \frac{1}{\Gamma(1/\gamma)} r_i^{\frac{1}{\gamma}-1} \exp\left(\frac{-r_i}{\gamma}\right) \;\text{ with } \mathbb{E}(r_i) = \psi_R = 1 \;\text{ and }\; \text{Var}(r_i) = \gamma\psi_R.$$

The log-likelihood for r_i is thus

$$\log(g(r_i)) = \sum_{i=1}^{n_i} \frac{\log r_i - r_i}{\gamma} - \frac{\log \gamma}{\gamma} - \log(\Gamma(1/\gamma)).$$

Referring to Eq. (21.4), $\lambda = \gamma$, $\theta_R = \log r_i = v_i$, and $b_R = \exp v_i$ so that $\log(g(r_i))$ is conjugate.

21.2.2 Bayesian Formulation

The Bayesian specifies a probability model for each stage of the hierarchy using corresponding covariates. Because there are no constraints on the means of the random effects, we return to the initial parameterization

$$l(\mu_{ij}) = \sum_{p=1}^{P} x_{pj}\beta_p + \beta_{0i}$$

where β_{0i} is a random effect.

1. Stage I. Conditional on the random effect, the outcomes Y_{ij} are independent and arise from a one parameter exponential distribution such that for cluster i,

$$y_{ij} \mid \boldsymbol{\beta}, \beta_{0i} \overset{\text{indep.}}{\sim} f(y_{ij} \mid \boldsymbol{\beta}, \beta_{0i}) \propto \prod_{j=1}^{n_i} \exp\left(\frac{y_{ij}\theta_{ij} - b(\theta_{ij}) + c(y_{ij})}{\phi}\right), \quad (21.5)$$

   where $\mathbb{E}(y_{ij} \mid \boldsymbol{\beta}, \beta_{0i}) = \mu_{ij}$, $\theta_{ij} = \theta(\mu_{ij})$, and $\text{Var}(Y_{ij} \mid \boldsymbol{\beta}, \beta_{0i}) = \phi V(\mu_{ij})$.
2. Stage II. The random effects, conditional on the *hyperparameters*[4], $\boldsymbol{\gamma}$, are exchangeable or partially exchangeable,[5] and follow a distribution from a one parameter exponential distribution proportional to

$$\prod_{i=1}^{I} \exp\left(\frac{\psi_B\theta_B(\beta_{0i}) - b_B(\theta_B(\beta_{0i}))}{\lambda}\right), \quad (21.6)$$

   where $l(\beta_{0i}) = \mathbf{w}_i\boldsymbol{\gamma}$, $\mathbb{E}(\beta_{0i} \mid \boldsymbol{\gamma}) = \psi_B$, $\text{Var}(\beta_{0i} \mid \boldsymbol{\gamma}) = \rho \text{V}(\psi_B)$, λ is a dispersion parameter, and where $\theta_B()$ and $b_B()$ are functions.
3. Stage III. The hyperparameters and Stage I/II parameters not varying by i arise from probability distributions $\boldsymbol{\gamma} \sim \pi_\gamma$; $\beta \sim \pi_\beta$; $\phi \sim \pi_\phi$.

The Stage II model need not be conjugate to the Stage I model–see Daniels and Gatsonis [80] who propose that β_{0i} comes from a t-distribution. As in the HLM, the conditional posterior mean of θ_{ij} can be expressed as

$$\mathbb{E}(\theta_{ij} \mid \beta_{0i}, D, y_{ij}) = S(D) \times l^{-1}(\mathbf{w}_i\boldsymbol{\gamma}) + (1 - S(D))\widehat{\theta}_{ij}(y_{ij}) \quad (21.7)$$

with $S(D)$, the shrinkage parameter introduced in the prior chapter that is constrained to lie in the interval (0, 1) and D are variance components.

[4] Hyperparameters are the parameters governing the Stage II distribution.
[5] The random effects are exchangeable within subgroups defined by the covariates $\mathbf{w}_i$.

21.2.2.1 Example: Normal Stage I and Normal Stage II Model

Representing the random effects by β_{0i} (rather than r_i), Stage II becomes

$$g(\beta_{0i}) \propto \prod_{i=1}^{I} \frac{\left(\beta_{0i}\mu_i - \frac{\mu_i}{2}\right)}{D} - \frac{1}{2}\left(\frac{\beta_{0i}^2}{D} + \log(2\pi)\right)$$

where $\mu_i = \mathbf{w}_i\boldsymbol{\gamma} = \mathbb{E}(\beta_{0i} \mid \boldsymbol{\gamma})$. Stage III is

$$\boldsymbol{\beta} \sim \pi_{\beta}; \boldsymbol{\gamma} \sim \pi_{\gamma}; \text{ and } D \sim \pi_D.$$

The difference between the frequentist and Bayesian approaches is the addition of distributions for all parameters. Of course, the interpretation of probability differs between the two frameworks, which we do not discuss here. There is a lengthy literature on the use of frequentist versus Bayesian inferential approaches that is beyond the scope of this textbook. We defer the discussion of how to make inferences to the next chapter and next describe some common examples of HGLMs.

21.3 Hierarchical Logistic Regression Model

Suppose Y_{ij} is a binary-valued patient-level outcome that assumes a value of 1 if an event occurs and 0 otherwise. A model for the probability that patient j treated at hospital i has the event has linear predictor

$$\log\left(\frac{\mu_{ij}}{1-\mu_{ij}}\right) = \log\left(\frac{\mathbb{P}(Y_{ij}=1 \mid \boldsymbol{\theta}_i, \boldsymbol{\phi}, \mathbf{x}_{ij})}{1-\mathbb{P}(Y_{ij}=1 \mid \boldsymbol{\theta}_i, \boldsymbol{\phi}, \mathbf{x}_{ij})}\right) = \sum_p \phi_p x_{pij} + \sum_q \theta_{qi} x_{qij},$$

where $\mu_{ij} = \mathbb{E}(Y_{ij} = 1 \mid \theta_i, \phi, \mathbf{x}_{ij})$ is the conditional probability of the event. The covariate effects and random effects are additive on the linear scale and multiplicative on the probability scale. Returning to the example in Volume 2, Chapter 20, "Introduction to Hierarchical Linear Models," suppose Y_{ij} is equal to 1 if the patient was satisfied with the care received and 0 otherwise. Let $\mathbf{x}_{ij}$ include patient age and severity at hospital admission and sex. Figure 21.1 provides a summary of the data for 1,977 patients treated at 20 hospitals presented earlier but uses a binary rather than continuous outcome. The proportion responding satisfied across all hospitals is 0.11 and ranges 10-fold, from 0.034 to 0.33.

A model for the probability that the jth patient treated at the ith hospital is satisfied with the care received could be

$$\begin{aligned} P(Y_{ij}=1 \mid \theta_i, \boldsymbol{\beta}, \mathbf{x}_{ij}) &\overset{indep.}{\sim} \text{Bernoulli}(p(\theta_i, \boldsymbol{\beta}, \mathbf{x})), \\ \text{logit}(p(\theta_i, \boldsymbol{\beta}, \mathbf{x}_{ij})) &= \theta_i + \beta_1 \text{Age}_{ij} + \beta_2 \text{Female}_{ij} + \beta_3 \text{Severity}_{ij}, \end{aligned} \tag{21.8}$$

where we permit only the intercept to vary across hospitals and $\phi = 1$. The regression coefficients are on the logit scale, which, when implementing Gelman and Hill's [26] *divide by four* rule, provides an upper bound of the change in the probability of outcome for a unit change in the covariate. The logit link also enables the estimation of odds ratios by exponentiating the regression coefficients. Thus, $\beta_2/4$ represents the change in the probability of satisfaction between females and males, and $\exp(\beta_2)$ represents the odds that a female is satisfied with care relative to the odds a male is satisfied. Because age and severity are continuous, $\exp(\beta_1)$ and $\exp(\beta_3)$ represent

Figure 21.1 Patient hospital satisfaction probabilities. Boxplots of patient age and severity at admission by satisfaction status, probability of satisfaction by sex, and scatterplot of proportion satisfied by hospital sample size for 1,977 patients treated at 20 hospitals.

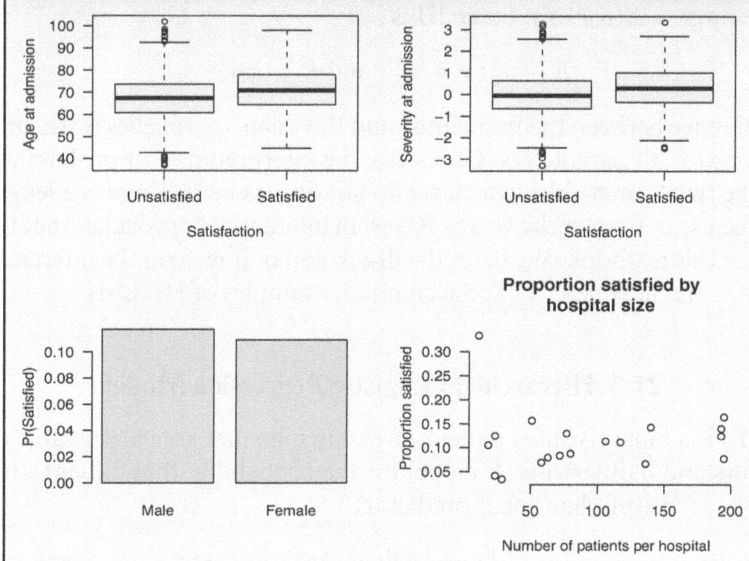

the odds of an increase of 1 year or 1 unit in age and severity, respectively, on being satisfied. In the Stage I model, there is no additive patient-specific error term as there was in the Stage I model for the HLM.

In the Stage II, the distribution for θ_i is $\theta_i \mid \mu, \tau^2 \overset{indep.}{\sim} N(\mu, \tau^2)$. The parameter τ^2 represents between-hospital variation in the log-odds of patient satisfaction, adjusting for patient sex, age, and severity at admission. As above, $\tau/4$ indicates the difference among hospitals on the probability scale. If $\tau^2 = 0$, then

$$\begin{aligned} \theta_{01} &= \theta_{02} = \cdots = \theta_{0I} = \theta \\ \text{so that } l(\mu_{ij}) &= \theta + \beta_1 \text{Age}_{ij} + \beta_2 \text{Female}_{ij} + \beta_3 \text{Severity}_{ij}, \end{aligned}$$

implying that any of the differences in the logits of satisfaction among hospitals is entirely due to hospital case-mix and Bernoulli random error. The conditional mean of the hospital random effects is

$$\mathbb{E}(\theta_i \mid \boldsymbol{\beta}, \tau, \mathbf{x}) = (1 - S_i)\hat{\theta}_i(y_{ij}) + S_i \text{logit}^{-1}(\mathbf{x}\boldsymbol{\beta}), \tag{21.9}$$

where $\hat{\theta}_i(y_{ij})$ is a function of the outcomes associated with provider i, y_{ij}, S_i is the shrinkage parameter, and $\text{logit}^{-1}()$ is the inverse logit function. As before, S_i lies in the interval (0,1). Thus, the expected outcome for the hospital, as in the linear model, is a compromise between an estimate using its data and one using a linear predictor.

Table 21.2 Estimated regression parameters.

	Logistic regression		Hierarchical regression	
Covariate	**Estimate**	**Standard error**	**Estimate**	**Standard error**
Intercept	NA	NA	−2.13	0.10
Age (centered), years	0.040	0.0074	0.040	0.0073
Female	−0.095	0.16	−0.11	0.16
Severity (centered)	0.36	0.074	0.35	0.073
Standard deviation				
$\hat{\tau}$	0		0.16	

Binary outcome is 1 if the patient is satisfied with the care received; otherwise 0. Higher values of the severity score correspond to sicker patients.

21.3.1 Adjustment for Patient Risk Factors

The linear predictor in the logistic regression model is

$$\text{logit}(P(Y_{ij} = 1) = \left(\sum_{i=1}^{I} \beta_{0i} I_{ij}\right) + \beta_1 \text{Age}_{ij} + \beta_2 \text{Female}_{ij} + \beta_3 \text{Severity}_{ij}$$

where, as before, we set $I_{ij} = 1$ if patient j was treated in hospital i and 0 otherwise. The model can be estimated in R using

```
glm(outcomes ~ factor(hosp.id) + cage + female + cseverity -1,
family=binomial(link=''logit''),data=lindata.set)
```

The estimated regression coefficients are reported in Table 21.2. Dividing the estimated regression coefficient of severity by 4 (0.36/4 = 0.09) suggests that an increase of 1 severity unit is associated with a 9% change in being satisfied. The association between females and satisfaction is not different from zero, and an increase of 1 year in age is associated with a 1% difference in satisfaction. The hierarchical logistic regression model is estimated using

```
glmer(outcomes ~ (1:hosp.id) + cage + female + cseverity,
family=binomial(link=''logit''), data=lindata.set)
```

which uses a generalized linear mixed model framework. The parameter estimates are also reported in Table 20.1. The qualitative interpretations of the regression coefficients do not change when compared to the logistic model when examining the risk-adjusted estimated coefficients derived from the hierarchical model. The between-hospital standard deviation is 0.16, indicating that hospitals differ by about 4% on the probability scale (divide by 4 rule).

21.3.2 Intraclass Correlation Coefficient

Intraclass correlation coefficients for binary data may be computed in a variety of ways. For instance, an analysis of variance (ANOVA) estimator (proposed for continuous data) has been used for the ICC. However, for rare events, this estimate could be negative. An alternative estimator for the ICC when modeling a binary outcome using a random-intercept only logistic regression model is

$$\hat{\rho} = \frac{\hat{\tau}^2}{\hat{\tau}^2 + \frac{\pi^2}{3}}. \tag{21.10}$$

The term $\frac{\pi^2}{3}$ arises from assuming an underlying continuous variable Y_{ij}^* such that $Y_{ij} = 1$ if $Y_{ij}^* > 0$ and

$$Y_{ij}^* = \sum_p \phi_p x_{pij} + \sum_q \theta_{qi} x_{qij} + \epsilon_{ij},$$

where ϵ_{ij} is assumed to have a logistic distribution with mean 0 and variance $\frac{\pi^2}{3}$. Using the estimate of τ^2 from the model adjusted for covariates yields an ICC = 0.007, indicating a weak provider signal.

21.3.3 Reliability

Another measure of the signal in provider profiling is interpreted as the correlation between the provider's true measure and the estimate of the measure. In the binary setting, each provider has its measure of reliability because reliability depends on between-provider variation, τ^2, the within-provider sample size, n_i, and the provider's true underlying outcome measure, p_i,

$$\text{Reliability} \quad r_i = \frac{\tau^2}{\tau^2 + \frac{p_i(1-p_i)}{n_i}}.$$

Thus, for a fixed value of τ^2 and n_i, reliability increases as p_i moves away from 0.50. For providers with true underlying event rates close to 0 or 1, reliability is high, whereas reliability is lowest among providers with rates near 0.50. Inter-unit reliability, discussed in Volume 2, Chapter 20, "Introduction to Hierarchical Linear Models," for the linear model varies only by n_i if we assume that $\sigma_i^2 = \frac{\sigma^2}{n_i}$. Increasing the provider sample size, therefore, increases reliability for both continuous and binary outcomes. However, in the continuous case, reliability would be the same across providers if sample sizes were equal, whereas in the binary setting, reliability would still vary among providers even if all providers had the same sample size.

21.3.4 Range in Variation

Interpretation of the variance component in the hierarchical logistic regression model can also be made on the logarithmic scale. As discussed in the prior chapter, the distance between the 97.5% and 2.5% log-odds ratios is $2 \times 1.96 \times \tau$ when $\theta_i \sim N(0, \tau^2)$. This, in turn, implies that the range in the ratio of odds ratios is $\exp(2 \times 1.96 \times \tau)$. Using the GLLM formulation in the example, $2 \times 1.96 \times \tau$ is the range in the hospital residuals. In the example, the range in odds ratios for the hospital residuals is 1.86.

21.3.5 Median Ratio of Random Provider Effects

An alternative summary of between-provider variation is the median ratio of the maximum to minimum provider effects of any pair of provider-specific odds ratios sampled from the random effects distribution. Under the assumption of Normality of the random effects with mean 0 and variance τ^2, the distribution of the absolute value of the difference between two randomly selected provider effects arises from a half normal distribution with mean 0. variance $2\tau^2$ that has a median at 1.09τ. On the odds ratio scale, reporting $\exp(1.09\tau)$ yields the median ratio for a pair of odds ratios. With $\hat{\tau} = 0.158$, the median ratio is 1.19.

21.4 Hierarchical Poisson Regression Model

Suppose Y_{ij} is the count of individuals undergoing coronary artery bypass grafting surgery in hospital j located in state i, and interests centers on characterizing geographic variation in surgical rates. Letting n_{ij} denote the number of individuals having a heart attack and treated at hospital j, state i, then

$$\mathbb{E}(Y_{ij} \mid \theta_i) = n_{ij}\mu_{ij} = n_{ij}\exp(\mathbf{x}_{ij}\boldsymbol{\beta} + \theta_i), \tag{21.11}$$

where $\mathbf{x}_{ij}$ denotes hospital characteristics, such as academic affiliation and nurse-to-bed ratio. Thus, the counts are assumed to arise from a Poisson distribution. Suppose the random effect, θ_i, arises from a Normal distribution

$$\theta_i = \mu + \omega_i \tag{21.12}$$

where ω_i is $N(0, \tau^2)$. State covariates, such as geographic region, race/ethnicity distribution of the state's adult population, managed care penetration, and uninsurance rates could be included. A Bayesian specification requires prior distributions for the remaining parameters, $\boldsymbol{\beta}$, μ, τ^2.

The variance component τ^2 characterizes between-state variation in surgical rates after accounting for patient characteristics. Another selection for the distribution of the random effects is the Gamma distribution, for example,

$$\theta \sim \text{Gamma}(\delta, \gamma) \;\; \delta > 0 \text{ and } \gamma > 0.$$

This distribution has mean $\delta\gamma$ and variance $\delta\gamma^2$. When δ is large, the Gamma distribution looks like the normal distribution. The rationale for the selection of the Gamma is made for computational convenience because the Gamma distribution is conjugate to the Poisson.

A frequentist approach to the same Poisson regression model re-expresses the mean as

$$\begin{aligned} \mathbb{E}(Y_{ij} \mid r_i) &= n_{ij}\mu_{ij};\; \log\mu_{ij} = \mathbf{x}_{ij}\boldsymbol{\beta} + \nu_i;\; \nu_i = \log r_i, && (21.13)\\ \mathbb{E}(r_i) &= 0 \text{ and } \text{Var}(r_i) = \tau^2. && (21.14) \end{aligned}$$

The random effects are additive on the log scale, but the Normal distribution is not conjugate to the Poisson. Using a Gamma distribution for the random effect, the mean is fixed

$$\mathbb{E}(r_i) = 1 \text{ and } \text{Var}(r_i) = \gamma. \tag{21.15}$$

Dispersion parameters can also be modelled (Box 21.1).

Box 21.1 Modeling the Stage I Dispersion Parameter

In both the frequentist and Bayesian approaches, a probability distribution for the Stage I dispersion parameter, ϕ, could be specified. In the frequentist setting, such models are denoted *double hierarchical generalized linear models* (DHGLM). For instance, using a link function, h, random and non-random effects may be used in a linear predictor,

$$h(\phi_{ij}) = \mathbf{x}^*_{ij}\boldsymbol{\gamma} + \mathbf{z}^*_{ij}\mathbf{b}_i.$$

In Volume 2, Chapter 20, for instance, the within-person standard deviation was permitted to vary by the person's sex and a random effect.

21.5 Provider-Specific Estimators

We define the expected outcome, ρ_i, for the ith provider conditional on the provider's random effects and the case-mix of the population it treated. In the binary outcome setting, the ATT has two components

$$\rho_i = \frac{1}{n_i}\sum_{j=1}^{n_i} E(Y_{ij} \mid \mathbf{x}_{ij}, \boldsymbol{\theta}_i, \phi) \text{ and } \rho_i^C = \frac{1}{n_i}\sum_{j=1}^{n_i}\int_{\boldsymbol{\theta}_i} E(Y_{ij} \mid \mathbf{x}_{ij}, \boldsymbol{\theta}_i, \phi, \boldsymbol{\alpha}) d\boldsymbol{\theta}_i \quad (21.16)$$

cannot be calculated in closed form, given the non-linearity of the model. The counterfactual outcomes for patients treated by provider i are obtained by averaging over the random effects of all providers, for example, the marginal distribution of Y_{ij}. Returning to the hierarchical logistic regression model for patient satisfaction,

$$\rho_i = \frac{1}{n_i}\sum_{j=1}^{n_i} \text{logit}^{-1}(\theta_i + \beta_1\text{Age}_{ij} + \beta_2\text{Female}_{ij} + \beta_3\text{Severity}_{ij}).$$

Unlike in the HLM,

$$\rho_i^C \neq \frac{1}{n_i}\sum_{j=1}^{n_i} \text{logit}^{-1}(\mu + \beta_1\text{Age}_{ij} + \beta_2\text{Female}_{ij} + \beta_3\text{Severity}_{ij}).$$

We use $\frac{1}{n_i}\sum_{j=1}^{n_i} \text{logit}^{-1}(\mu + \beta_1\text{Age}_{ij} + \beta_2\text{Female}_{ij} + \beta_3\text{Severity}_{ij})$ to define a counterfactual outcome when it is a close approximation to the marginal distribution. As in the prior chapter, functions of $\widehat{\rho}_i$ and $\widehat{\rho}_i^C$ may be used to infer the quality of provider i.

Figure 21.2 displays the hospital residuals obtained from the patient satisfaction data estimated using the `glmer` function. Exponentiating $\widehat{\omega}_i$ yields the estimated odds of the outcome at the ith hospital *relative* to the odds of the outcome at a hospital with $\omega_i = 0$ ("average" residual of 0) for patients having the *same covariate* values, for example,

$$\begin{aligned} \text{If } \text{logit}(p_{ij} \mid \omega_i) &= \mu + \omega_i + \beta_1\text{Age}_{ij} + \beta_2\text{Female}_{ij} + \beta_3\text{Severity}_{ij} \\ \text{then } d_i &= \text{logit}(p_{ij} \mid \omega = \omega_i) - \text{logit}(p_{ij} \mid \omega = 0) = \omega_i. \end{aligned}$$

The figure indicates that the hospital residuals ranged from -0.13 to 0.17, with the smallest and largest values, both linked with hospitals having more than 190 patients. The corresponding odds ratios are 0.88 and 1.19, representing the odds

Figure 21.2 Hospital residuals, satisfaction example. Estimated residuals on the logit scale (x-axis) are plotted against the hospital sample size (y-axis).

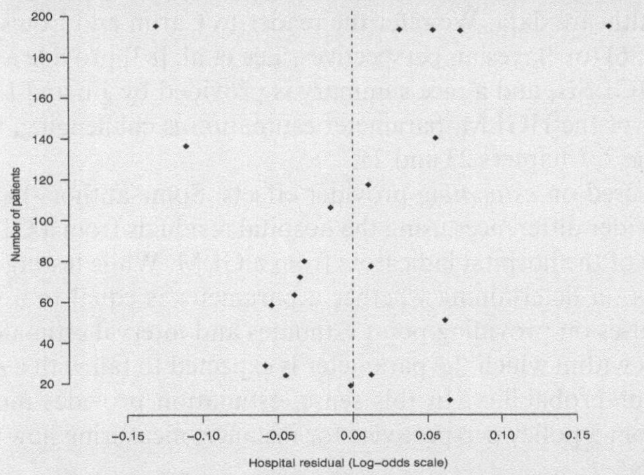

Box 21.2 "Observed" to "expected" outcome.

Assuming Y_{ij} is a binary outcome for the jth subject treated by provider i such that

$$Y_{ij} \overset{ind}{\sim} \text{Bern}(p_{ij}(\mathbf{X})) \text{ where } \text{logit}(p_{ij}(\mathbf{X})) = \theta_{0i} + \boldsymbol{\alpha}'\mathbf{X}_{ij} \text{ and } \theta_{0i} \sim N(\mu, \tau^2).$$

The potential outcome rate for provider i is

$$\rho_i^C = \frac{1}{n_i}\sum_{j=1}^{n_i} \text{logit}^{-1}\left(\mu + \boldsymbol{\alpha}'\mathbf{X}_{ij}\right). \tag{21.17}$$

Rather than the observed rate, $Y_i = \frac{1}{n_i}\sum_j Y_{ij}$ as described in Box 19.1 (Volume 2, Chapter 19, "A Causal Inference Framework"), use

$$\rho_i = \frac{1}{n_i}\sum_{j=1}^{n_i} \text{logit}^{-1}\left(\theta_{0i} + \boldsymbol{\alpha}'\mathbf{X}_{ij}\right) \tag{21.18}$$

so that the causal parameter for provider i is

$$\frac{\rho_i}{\rho_i^C} = \frac{\sum_{j=1}^{n_i} \text{logit}^{-1}\left(\theta_{0i} + \hat{\boldsymbol{\alpha}}'\mathbf{X}_{ij}\right)}{\sum_{j=1}^{n_i} \text{logit}^{-1}\left(\mu + \hat{\boldsymbol{\alpha}}'\mathbf{X}_{ij}\right)}. \tag{21.19}$$

Values larger than 1 indicate higher-than-expected outcomes and values less than 1 indicate lower-than-expected outcomes.

of being satisfied with the care delivered for each hospital relative to an average hospital treating identical patients.

Unfortunately, odds ratios are not on a scale with which most consumers of profiling information are familiar or desire. Of more direct interest are $\rho_i - \rho_i^C$ representing risk differences or $\frac{\rho_i}{\rho_i^C}$ (see Box 21.2).

21.6 Summary

The literature on generalized linear models is extensive. The interested reader should refer to the text authored by McCullagh [81]. Like GLMs, hierarchical generalized linear models accommodate a broad family of densities frequently utilized in the analysis of healthcare data. We refer the reader to Carlin and Louis [82] and Gelman and Hill [26] for Bayesian perspectives. Lee et al. [83] provide a non-Bayesian treatment of HGLMs, and a nice summary is provided by Jin and Lee [84]. Given the complexity of the HGLM, parameter estimation is challenging, and this is the topic of Volume 2, Chapters 23 and 24.

We have focused on *estimating* provider effects. Some authors have focused on *testing* for provider differences using the hospital residuals from a GLMM or using the coefficients of the hospital indicators from a GLM. While testing is always possible, it focuses on determining whether a parameter is equal to a specific value; estimation focuses on providing point estimates and interval estimates that yield a range of values within which the parameter is expected to fall with a specific degree of confidence or probability. In this sense, estimation provides more actionable information from a policy perspective—for instance, measuring how far a provider is from its peers.

Appendix: Bayesian GLMs

A Bayesian approach to GLMs may also be adopted by considering classes of priors for exponential family models. Assume $\phi = 1$ as is the case for the binomial and Poisson distributions. The exponential family density is thus written as

$$p(y \mid \theta) = \exp\{y\theta - b(\theta) + c(y)\}\,. \tag{21.20}$$

Theorem. Suppose $p(y \mid \theta)$ is given by (21.20). If the prior distribution for θ is of the form

$$\pi(\theta) \;\propto\; \exp\{a_0(\theta y_0 - b(\theta))\}, \tag{21.21}$$

where (a_0, y_0) are specified hyperparameters, then $\pi(\theta)$ is a conjugate prior[6] for θ, which indexes the exponential family $p(y \mid \theta)$.

Proof: Denote the prior distribution in (21.21) by $D(a_0, y_0)$ so that the prior is $\theta \sim D(a_0, y_0) \Rightarrow \pi(\theta) \;\propto\; \exp[a_0(\theta y_0 - b(\theta))]$. We want to show that the posterior distribution $\theta \mid y$ is also of type D.

$$\begin{aligned} p(\theta \mid y) &\propto p(y \mid \theta)\, \pi(\theta) \\ &\propto \exp[y\theta - b(\theta)]\exp[a_0(\theta y_0 - b(\theta))] \\ &= \exp[\theta(y + a_0 y_0) - (a_0 + 1)\, b(\theta)] \\ &= \exp\left[(a_0 + 1)\left\{\theta\left(\frac{y + a_0 y_0}{a_0 + 1}\right) - b(\theta)\right\}\right]. \end{aligned}$$

[6] Conjugate priors are proper priors by definition.

So $\theta \mid y \sim D\left(a_0+1,\ \frac{y+a_0y_0}{a_0+1}\right)$.

The posterior distribution has hyperparameters of the form $\left(a_0+1,\ \frac{y+a_0y_0}{a_0+1}\right)$ where

$$\frac{y+a_0y_0}{a_0+1}=\left(\frac{1}{a_0+1}\right)y+\left(\frac{a_0}{a_0+1}\right)y_0$$

is a weighted average of the data and the prior parameter y_0, with the weights being defined by a_0. Additionally, the parameter a_0 is updated to a_0+1 in going from the prior distribution of θ to the posterior after the collection of 1 observation y. With n i.i.d. observations $y_1,\ldots,y_n$, having

$$p(y_i \mid \theta)=\exp\{y_i\theta-b(\theta)+c(y_i)\} \quad \text{and} \quad \pi(\theta)\ \propto\ \exp[a_0(y_0\theta-b(\theta))],$$

$$\begin{aligned}\text{then,}\ \ p(\theta \mid y) &\propto \prod_{i=1}^{n} p(y_i \mid \theta)\,\pi(\theta)\\ &\propto \exp\{\theta\,\Sigma y_i-n\,b(\theta)\}\ \exp[a_0(\theta y_0-b(\theta))]\\ &\propto \exp\left\{(n+a_0)\left(\theta\left(\frac{n\bar{y}+a_0y_0}{n+a_0}\right)-b(\theta)\right)\right\}.\end{aligned}$$

$$\text{So } \theta \mid y \sim D\left(n+a_0,\ \frac{n\bar{y}+a_0y_0}{n+a_0}\right).$$

□

Example: Normal Model

Suppose $y \sim N(\mu, 1)$. In this case, we have $\theta=\mu,\ \ b(\theta)=\frac{\theta^2}{2}$ so

$$\text{Likelihood: } p(y \mid \theta)\ \propto\ \exp\left[-\frac{1}{2}(y-\theta)^2\right]$$

$$\begin{aligned}\text{Prior } \pi(\theta) &\propto \exp[a_0(\theta y_0-b(\theta))]=\exp\left[a_0\left(\theta y_0-\frac{\theta^2}{2}\right)\right]\\ &\propto \exp\left[-\frac{a_0}{2}(\theta-y_0)^2\right].\end{aligned}$$

Thus, $\theta \sim N(y_0, a_0^{-1})$ is the conjugate prior, where $-\infty < y_0 < \infty,\ a_0 > 0$.

Example: Binomial Model

Suppose $y \sim \text{Binomial}(1, p)$. In this case, we have $p=\frac{e^\theta}{1+e^\theta},\ \ b(\theta)=\log(1+e^\theta)$ so the

$$\begin{aligned}
\text{Likelihood}: \ p(y \mid \theta) &\propto \exp[y\theta - \log(1+e^{\theta})] \\
\text{Prior:} \ \pi(\theta) &\propto \exp[a_0(\theta y_0 - b(\theta))] \\
&= \exp[a_0\left(\theta y_0 - \log\left(1+e^{\theta}\right)\right)] \\
&= \frac{\exp(a_0 y_0 \theta)}{(1+\exp(\theta))^{a_0}} \\
&= \left(\frac{\exp(\theta)}{1+\exp(\theta)}\right)^{a_0 y_0} \left(\frac{1}{1+\exp(\theta)}\right)^{a_0(1-y_0)}
\end{aligned}$$

$$\text{Therefore } \pi(\theta) \propto \left(\frac{\exp(\theta)}{1+\exp(\theta)}\right)^{a_0 y_0} \left(\frac{1}{1+\exp(\theta)}\right)^{a_0(1-y_0)} .$$

This prior distribution is equivalent to a Beta prior distribution for θ. To see this, let $u = \frac{\exp(\theta)}{1+\exp(\theta)}$, $1-u = \frac{1}{1+\exp(\theta)}$.

$$\frac{du}{d\theta} = \frac{\exp(\theta)}{(1+\exp(\theta))^2} = u(1-u) .$$

$$\begin{aligned}
\pi(u) &\propto u^{a_0 y_0}(1-u)^{a_0(1-y_0)} \left(u^{-1}(1-u)^{-1}\right) \\
&= u^{a_0 y_0 - 1}(1-u)^{a_0(1-y_0)-1} .
\end{aligned}$$

Thus $u \sim \text{beta}(a_0 y_0, a_0(1-y_0))$ where $u = \frac{\exp(\theta)}{1+\exp(\theta)}$, $a_0 > 0$, $0 < y_0 < 1$. Therefore, the conjugate prior for the binomial family is a Beta distribution.

CHAPTER TWENTY-TWO

Composite Measures and Multiple Outcomes

Volume 1, Chapter 11, "Composite Performance Measures," introduced composite healthcare performance measures, describing their use in other fields, as well as various conceptual frameworks proposed by investigators. In this chapter, we adopt a psychometric framework for measuring quality. Our premise is that the multiple individual observed process and outcome measures provide information about an underlying quality construct or possibly several underlying constructs. These constructs are unobserved and sometimes are referred to as latent variables. Given most quality metrics are categorical, we first introduce Item Response Theory Models (IRT). These models may be thought of as factor analysis models for discrete data. We then move to approaches to modeling *multiple* outcomes where the focus is on each outcome. Modeling approaches for responses that consist of both discrete and continuous metrics, denoted *mixed outcomes*, are discussed. There are several statistical approaches for modeling mixed outcomes simultaneously—some focus on making inferences about the underlying latent constructs, and others focus on the individual outcomes, treating the correlation among the outcomes as nuisance parameters. For instance, interest may center on comparing whether quality metrics differ between patients whose care is managed and patients whose care is not managed. In this setting, the researcher is interested in the specific associations of managed care with each outcome. When the outcomes are mixed, the main challenge is identifying a suitable multivariate distribution. To avoid specifying the joint distribution of the mixed outcomes directly, three general approaches have been proposed: factorizing the joint likelihood, introducing a latent variable that connects the mixed outcomes, or modeling each outcome separately and then using a working correlation to account for the dependence among the outcomes.

The question dealt with in this chapter is how to use individual metrics, possibly measured on different scales, to assess quality of care at both the patient and provider levels.

22.1 Opportunity Scoring

Table 22.1a (hospitals $\geqslant$ 30 person-measures) and Table 22.1b (all hospitals), first introduced in Volume 1, Chapter 2, "Conceptual Models," describe multiple process metrics for pneumonia patients treated at US hospitals. The summary

Table 22.1a Process measures for community acquired pneumonia across US hospitals ⩾ 30 person-measures.

Metric	No. of hospitals	% Receiving therapy
Oxygenation assessment	3,714	97.8
Pneumococcal vaccination	3,710	43.4
Blood culture before first antibiotic	2,904	82.0
Smoking cessation advice	2,815	60.8
Antibiotics within 4 hours of arrival	3,713	72.3
Opportunity score	3,714	76.3

Oxygenation assessment = blood oxygenation assessment within 24 hours of arrival; pneumococcal vaccination = patients aged ⩾ 65 screened for vaccination status and vaccinated if appropriate; blood culture before first antibiotic = blood culture specimen collected before receipt of antibiotics; adult smoking cessation advice/counseling = smoking cessation advice or counseling for smokers; = antibiotics < 4 hours of hospital arrival = receipt of an initial dose of antibiotic within 4 hours of arrival to the hospital.

Table 22.1b Process measures for community acquired pneumonia across all hospitals.

Metric	No. of hospitals	% Receiving therapy
Oxygenation assessment	3,898	97.6
Pneumococcal vaccination	3,871	42.9
Blood culture before first antibiotic	2,970	81.9
Smoking cessation advice	2,852	60.7
Antibiotics within 4 hours of arrival	3,894	72.4
Opportunity score	3,899	76.1

See note in Table 22.1a.

measure, an *opportunity score*, was obtained by dividing the sum of all eligible person-measures where recommended care was provided by the sum of all eligible person-measures. Information is provided for all hospitals (22.1b) as well as for hospitals in which there were at least 30 person-measures reported (Table 22.1a). This latter constraint is used by the Centers for Medicare and Medicaid Services when computing a hospital's composite score for some of their programs.

Examination of the table reveals that oxygenation assessment is undertaken on virtually all pneumonia patients, whereas few eligible patients received a pneumococcal vaccination. Not all hospitals had patients for some measures, as can be inferred from the changing number of hospitals for each quality metric.

Let Y_{kji} denote the outcome associated with quality metric i for individual j treated by provider k. We refer to the quality metrics as *items*. Response options for the items are binary, with a value of 1 corresponding to receiving the needed service and 0 indicating otherwise. We assume there are I items, n_k individuals treated by provider k, and K providers. The total number of individuals is $N = \sum_{k=1}^{K} n_k$. Not all metrics will apply to an individual, so we let n_{kj} denote the number of measures for which individual j is eligible. In the example, there are $I = 5$ items for each patient, and $K = 3,899$ hospitals.

The commonly employed estimators of quality received by individual j treated by provider k and of provider k's quality are, respectively,

$$\hat{\theta}_{kj} = \bar{Y}_{kj\cdot} = \frac{1}{n_{kj}} \sum_{i=1}^{n_{kj}} Y_{kji} \text{ and } \hat{\theta}_k = \bar{Y}_{k\cdot\cdot} = \frac{1}{n_k} \sum_{j=1}^{n_k} \hat{\theta}_{kj}. \tag{22.1}$$

Weights based on the perceived importance of a metric are sometimes used (see Volume 1, Chapter 11, "Composite Performance Measures"), although there is often controversy among stakeholders for the selected values. The estimator $\hat{\theta}_k$ is the opportunity score. Using these approaches, estimators for specific patient subgroups are typically determined by averaging within subgroups. For instance, the black-white quality disparity estimator associated with the kth provider is

$$\frac{1}{\sum_{j=1} x_{kj}} \sum_{j=1}^{n_k} \hat{\theta}_{kj} x_{kj} - \frac{1}{n_k - \sum_{j=1}^{n_k} x_{kj}} \sum_{j=1}^{n_k} \hat{\theta}_{kj}(1 - x_{kj}),$$

where $x_{kj} = 1$ if the individual is black and 0 if the individual is white.

While this approach is simple to interpret and easy to calculate, there are several problems. The first obvious issue is that the approach assumes all metrics use the same response scale, which sometimes is unlikely. Continuous or count outcomes could be converted to binary responses, although information for discriminating across quality may be lost. Second, even when the metrics use the same scale, the underlying frequency of each metric may differ. In this situation, the optimal (in terms of variance) algorithm for pooling information depends upon the type of measurement error present, which in turn depends on the underlying frequency of the metric. Third, pooling algorithms are not clearly defined if some items are missing (different from not applicable). The fourth problem relates to the various levels of correlation that have been ignored when using the opportunity score. For each individual, there are multiple related responses measured. Moreover, within each provider, observations between two individuals are correlated—in fact, this reflects the basis for assessing providers. While accounting for multiple measurements per person and provider could be achieved through the deployment of a robust variance estimator, the need for provider-specific estimates and functions of the estimates suggests the use of a hierarchical model.

22.2 Item Response Theory Model for Categorical Outcomes

The underlying premise in an item response theory (IRT) model is that each observed quality metric is a manifestation of a single or a few latent variables, and the latent variables are the primary focus of inference. These variables quantify the underlying quality received by a patient and delivered by providers. Observed responses for each quality metric are linked through these latent constructs. The quality constructs could differ between patient groups, in which case a *structural model* for the latent variables would specify patient-level covariates. Between-provider variation is also introduced in the structural model.

Ignoring the provider index, k, for now, assuming a dichotomous item (quality indicator) and a single latent variable, a commonly used model is the *2-Parameter Logistic (2PL)* model defined as

$$P(Y_{ji} = 1 \mid \theta_j) = \frac{\exp(a_i(\theta_j - b_i))}{1 + \exp(a_i(\theta_j - b_i))}. \tag{22.2}$$

The term θ_j is the underlying latent trait (quality in our setting), a_i is an item discrimination parameter, and b_i is an item difficulty parameter. These names come from the field of education where, for instance, items are math questions and the latent trait is math ability. The IRT model connects binary observations to item-specific parameters and a latent trait. The IRT model differs from the common factor model in that factor models assume the observed measurements are continuous so that the measurement error is additive (Box 22.1). The quality metrics are scored so that values of 1 correspond to better quality compared to values of 0. The larger the value of a_i, the more discriminating the latent trait item i is. If $a_1 = a_2 = \cdots a_I = 1$, then the IRT model has a random intercept only (referred to as a *Rasch* model), and $\bar{Y}_{\cdot kj}$ is a sufficient statistic for θ_j conditional on b_i. Thus, it is only when the item discrimination parameters are equal that an unweighted sum of the binary metrics, as defined in Eq. (22.1), is suitable for estimating the latent construct. If some of the discrimination parameters differ, then the *pattern* of outcomes, rather than the total or average outcome, is important. The link function is the logit link in Eq. (22.2), although a probit link would work as well, and we use it in the next example.

Person characteristics are linked to the latent trait using a *structural* model,

$$\theta_j = \mathbf{X}_j^\top \gamma + \epsilon_j \tag{22.3}$$

where $\mathbf{X}_j$ is a vector of person variables. The covariates affect the response only through the latent variable.

Box 22.1 The common factor model

If Y_{ji} is the response to the ith item by person j, a common factor model is defined by

$$Y_{ji} = \lambda_i \theta_j + \epsilon_{ji},$$

where θ_j represents the latent construct for subject j, λ_i is a factor loading for item i, and ϵ_{ji} is a measurement error and define $\text{Var}(\theta_j) = \tau^2$ and $\text{Var}(\epsilon_i) = \sigma_i^2$. It is assumed that θ_j is independent of ϵ_{ji}. To identify the model, the variance of the latent trait is fixed, $\tau^2 = 1$, often assuming $\theta_j \sim N(0, 1)$, or a loading is set to 1, $\lambda_1 = 1$. This is referred to as factor standardization in the first case and anchoring in the second case.

22.2.1 Pneumonia Example

Table 22.2 provides the item parameter estimates and corresponding 95% confidence intervals for the 5 pneumonia quality metrics in Table 22.1a. The estimates are based on a 2-Parameter Probit model. Figure 22.1 displays the opportunity scores and the estimated latent construct from the model. The right-hand plot in Figure 22.1 presents the distribution of the opportunity scores using the pneumonia metrics. The histogram is left-skewed with some hospitals having a low opportunity score, below 60. The left-hand plot is an *Item Characteristic Curve* that plots the relationship of each quality metric on the probability scale with the latent quality construct obtained from the model. The latent construct is scaled as an N(0,1) random variable for identifiability of the model parameters. Higher values of the latent construct correspond to better pneumonia care quality. The discrimination parameters, a_i, drive the slope of each ICC, while the difficulty parameters, b_i, indicate

Table 22.2 Item parameter estimates for community acquired pneumonia across US hospitals. 2-Parameter Probit Model.

Metric	$\hat{a}_i$	95% CI	$\hat{b}_i$	95% CI
Oxygenation assessment	0.28	(0.27,0.30)	−2.20	(−2.22,−2.19)
Pneumococcal vaccination	0.89	(0.87,0.91)	0.25	(0.22,0.28)
Blood culture before first antibiotic	0.16	(0.16,0.17)	−0.51	(−0.52,−0.51)
Smoking cessation advice	0.37	(0.35,0.39)	−0.34	(−0.36,−0.32)
Antibiotics within 4 hours of arrival	0.19	(0.08,0.10)	−0.93	(−0.94,−0.92)

Figure 22.1 Community acquired pneumonia hospital quality. Latent quality scores estimated using a 2-Parameter Logistic model.

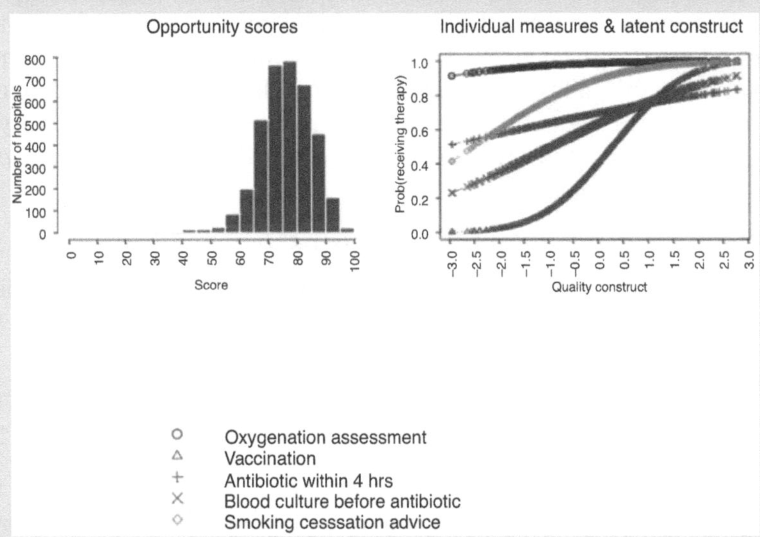

where each curve starts on the y-axis. Oxygenation assessment was employed on virtually everyone, and this is reflected by (1) the high probabilities across the range of quality and (2) the horizontal shape of the ICC. This conveys that this particular metric is not discriminating well across different ranges of latent quality. The estimate of b_i is the smallest of the 5 measures. In contrast, vaccination covers the full range of the y-axis and does appear to discriminate between low pneumonia care quality (quality < -1.0) and higher quality (quality > 1.0).[1]

For quality measures having polytomous responses, a nominal IRT model

$$P(Y_{ji} = p \mid \theta_j) = \frac{\exp(a_i^p(\theta_j - b_i^p))}{\sum_s \exp(a_i^s(\theta_j - b_i^s))} \tag{22.4}$$

where quality metric i has response options $p = 0, 1, \ldots, P_i - 1$ is often estimated. In this model, item parameters are specific to the response options. IRT models for ordinal data as well as additional model features, such as a guessing parameter, have been developed and used extensively outside of the healthcare quality setting. Baker [85] provides a detailed technical discussion of IRT models.

22.2.2 Hierarchical IRT Models

The IRT model itself is, of course, a hierarchical model with items nested within subjects. Further levels of clustering are natural, as in our setting, where individuals are also nested within providers. The model in Eq. (22.2) becomes

$$P(Y_{kji} = 1 \mid \theta_{kj}) = \frac{\exp(a_i(\theta_{kj} - b_i))}{1 + \exp(a_i(\theta_{kj} - b_i))}, \tag{22.5}$$

where the latent trait, θ_{kj}, is indexed by provider k. Person-level characteristics are included using a *structural model* that links the latent trait to person characteristics,

$$\text{Stage I:} \quad \theta_{kj} = \mathbf{X}_{kj}^{\top}\boldsymbol{\gamma}_k + \delta_{kj}, \tag{22.6}$$

where the associations between the latent trait and person characteristics may vary across providers as indicated by the subscript k on $\boldsymbol{\gamma}$. The term δ_{kj} represents residual variation in quality provided to an individual not already accounted for by person covariates. Not all person-level covariate effects need to vary across providers; a random intercept may be sufficient. To permit between-provider variation, Stage III becomes

$$\text{Stage II:} \quad \boldsymbol{\gamma}_k = \boldsymbol{\mu} + \boldsymbol{\epsilon}_k. \tag{22.7}$$

The parameter vector $\boldsymbol{\gamma}_k$ characterizes covariate effects for each provider. It is assumed $\mathbb{E}(\delta_{kj}) = 0$, $\text{Var}(\delta_{kj}) = \sigma^2$, $\mathbb{E}(\boldsymbol{\epsilon}_k) = \mathbf{0}$, and $\text{Var}(\boldsymbol{\epsilon}_k) = \mathbf{T}$.

[1] We note that because data were unavailable at the patient level, variation attributed to the patient has been ignored.

22.2.2.1 CHF Example

He et al. [86] examined the distribution of 3399 hospital congestive heart failure (CHF) quality scores across census regions and states (Table 22.3a). Four binary-valued process metrics were measured at each hospital: (a) if the patient was discharged with instructions; (b) if left ventricular function was assessed; (c) for patients with left ventricular systolic dysfunction, if an angiotensin-converting enzyme or an angiotensin receptor blocker was prescribed; and (d) for current smokers, if smoking cessation counseling was given. There is some variability among the census regions, with the Midwest and the Northeast having the highest scores compared to the other parts of the country. A 2-Parameter Probit model was used to link the process measures to latent quality, and a structural model linked latent quality to regions and states,

$$\begin{aligned} Y_{skji} &\sim \text{Binomial}(n_{ski}, p_{ski}), \\ \text{probit}(p_{ski} \mid \theta_{sk}) &= \frac{\exp(a_i(\theta_{sk} - b_i))}{1 + \exp(a_i(\theta_{sk} - b_i))} \\ \text{and } \theta_{sk} &= \beta_r + \gamma_s + \epsilon_{sk}. \end{aligned}$$

In the model, $Y_{skji} = 1$ for each patient j having metric i met in hospital k located in state s and 0 otherwise, and n_{ski} denotes the number of patients eligible for metric i; θ_{sk} is the quality of hospital k located in state s; β_r represents a fixed region effect quantifying the deviation of the region's average hospital quality from the national average; γ_s is a state random effect, and ϵ_{sk} is residual hospital-level variation. The

Table 22.3a Congestive heart failure hospital quality. Scores are based on 4 process measures.

Area	No. of hospitals	Opportunity score	Percentiles (2.5%, 97.5%)
National	3,399	0.77	(0.397, 0.972)
Midwest	874	0.79	(0.407, 0.983)
Northeast	557	0.80	(0.510, 0.971)
South	1,377	0.75	(0.347, 0.970)
West	591	0.73	(0.380, 0.956)

Table 22.3b Congestive heart failure hospital quality. Hierarchical 2-PL model. Scores are based on 4 process measures

Source	Variance	Estimate	% Variation explained
Region	$\frac{\sum_r n_r \beta_r^2}{N-1}$	0.053	4.7
State	τ^2	0.072	6.4
Hospital	σ^2	1	88.9

Figure 22.2 Hospital composite quality scores for CHF care. Latent quality scores were estimated using a 2-Parameter Logistic model, with no adjustment for region or state.

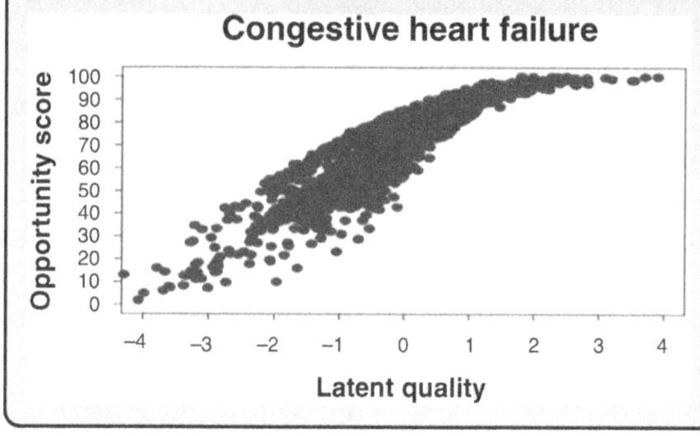

model assumes $\gamma_s \sim N(0, \tau^2)$, $\epsilon_{sk} \sim N(0, 1)$, and $\sum_r \beta_r = 0$. The last two assumptions are required for identifiability, which we discuss below and ensure that the average quality is 0 on the latent scale. The primary goal is to determine the extent of geographic variability in CHF hospital quality.

Figure 22.2 compares the hospital opportunity scores and the latent trait. The two composite scores are related, although differences are larger at the lower end of both scales. The primary reason for the differences at the lower end can be attributed to the number of measures contributed by each hospital. Hospitals with fewer measures tend to get higher opportunity scores because all measures are weighted equally—that is, there is no difference in the opportunity score between "easy to achieve" and "difficult to achieve" quality measures.

Table 22.3b partitions the variation in hospital quality into region, state, and hospital. More than 10% of the total variation in CHF quality is due to the location of hospitals, with 6% attributed to state. Summaries of the various parameters can be used to characterize state-specific quality. For instance,

$$P\left(\bar{\theta}_s = \frac{1}{n_s}\sum_{k=1}^{n_s}\theta_{sk} > 0\right)$$

represents the probability that average quality in state s is better than the national average, where n_s denotes the number of hospitals in state s. Large probabilities indicate that the state has better-than-average hospital quality. Determination of the expected fraction of higher-quality hospitals within each state could be operationalized using

$$\pi_{sk,\xi_{0.90}} = P(\theta_{sk} > \xi_{0.90} \mid \mathbf{Y}) = \frac{1}{n_s}\sum_{k=1}^{n_s}\pi_{sk,\xi_{0.90}},$$

where $\xi_{0.90}$ is the 90th percentile of the distribution of the θ_{sk}s across all states. Like the pneumonia example, data were only available at the hospital level, implying that correlation within patients among the repeated quality metrics has not been accounted for.

22.2.3 Assumptions

The IRT models assume that the responses between individuals are independent and conditional on the individual's latent trait, and responses within an individual are independent. Tests of conditional independence of the items include the likelihood ratio statistic based on determining the difference between the observed and model-predicted item responses from each item pair's contingency table [87]. The Q_3 [88] measures the correlation between the deviation of the observed and model-predicted item scores for each item. As in the usual hierarchical model, we assume that observations between individuals treated by the same provider are conditionally independent given the provider's random latent trait.

Assumptions about the variance components, such as a constant variance, σ^2 for δ^2_{kj}, require assessment. Given that the error terms are on the structural model, a comparison of observed versus predicted values may reveal problems.

22.2.4 Multidimensional Multilevel Quality Measurement

Thus far, the examples included only a few quality metrics so that only one latent trait is identifiable by the data. If more metrics are available, more than one latent construct may be identified. In this case, there are various modeling options, each depending on what is hypothesized about quality. Suppose interest centers on assessing quality of care as a general construct, denoted by ξ_j, and there are D domains, represented by θ_{kjd} for $d = 1, \ldots, D$. Then the structural model (Stage II) becomes

$$\theta_{kjd} = \lambda_d \xi_{kj} + \omega_{kjd}. \tag{22.8}$$

In this model, the domain-specific quality construct is linearly related to the general quality construct and an error term. The error term represents domain-specific quality not captured by ξ_{kj} and has $\text{Var}(\omega_{kjd}) = \sigma^2_{\omega_{kd}}$. Typically $\mathbb{E}(\omega_{kjd}\ \omega_{kjd*}) = 0$ for $d \neq d*$. This model provides an *overall* quality estimate that can be used to infer provider quality. The general construct is next modeled as

$$\xi_{kj} = \mathbf{X}_{kj}^{\top} \boldsymbol{\gamma}_k + \delta_{kj} \text{ where } \boldsymbol{\gamma}_k = \boldsymbol{\mu} + \boldsymbol{\epsilon}_k.$$

Alternatively, one could assume there are D uncorrelated constructs with

$$\theta_{kjd} = \mathbf{X}_{kjd}^{\top} \boldsymbol{\gamma}_{kd} + \delta_{kjd}. \tag{22.9}$$

Unlike the model in Eq. (22.8), there is no specific structure imposed on the constructs, and person-specific covariates can be domain-specific. When the constructs are uncorrelated, each would be estimated separately using a hierarchical approach. If and how to combine the individual constructs to arrive at an *overall* construct would be up to the researcher.

22.2.5 Identifiability

In non-hierarchical IRT models, the most common approach to identify the model parameters is to assume the latent construct arises from an $N(0, 1)$ distribution.

When adding additional structure to the data, such as a provider-level effect, the latent construct is a sum of variance components. Assume a 2PL model with latent trait θ_{kj} without any person-level covariates. Combining Stages III and II yields

$$\theta_{kj} = \delta_{kj} + \epsilon_k.$$

The scale of the latent dimension is the sum of two variance components, so fixing this to be one may not be sensible. In the hierarchical model setting, a common strategy sets one $a_i = 1$ and one $b_i = 0$. If covariates are included, then additional restrictions are required.

22.3 Latent Variable Models for Mixed Outcomes

While the majority of quality metrics are categorical, some metrics may be measured on a continuous scale. To model the multiple outcomes simultaneously, like the IRT model, a latent variable is introduced. To begin, consider just two outcomes, one binary and one continuous, and ignore provider clustering for now. Let Y_j^c and Y_j^b denote the continuous and binary outcomes for person j and $\mathbf{X}_j$, a vector of covariates. Assume $\text{Var}(Y_j^c) = \sigma^2$ and let

$$Y_j^b = \begin{cases} 1 & Y_j^{b*} \leqslant 0, \\ 0 & Y_j^{b*} > 0, \end{cases}$$

where Y_j^{b*} is an unobserved normally distributed variable that generates the binary variable. To link the two outcomes, Sammel et al. [89] suggested the probit link for the binary outcome and introduced a person-specific latent variable, θ_j

$$\text{probit}(P(Y_j^b = 1 \mid \theta_j)) = b_b + a_b\theta_j, \tag{22.10}$$

$$Y_j^c \mid \theta_j = b_c + a_c\theta_j + \epsilon_j, \tag{22.11}$$

where $\epsilon_j \sim N(0, \sigma^2)$. The structural model is

$$\theta_j = \mathbf{X}_j^T\gamma + \delta_j;\ \delta_j \sim N(0, 1). \tag{22.12}$$

Because this model is sensitive to model misspecification, Armando et al. (2009) proposed a different model. Letting $\mathbf{X}_j^c$ and $\mathbf{X}_j^b$ represent covariates thought to be related to the continuous and binary outcomes, then

$$\text{probit}(P(Y_j^b = 1 \mid \theta_j)) = \mathbf{x}_j^b\boldsymbol{\beta}^b + \theta_j, \tag{22.13}$$

$$Y_j^c \mid \theta_j = \mathbf{x}_j^c\boldsymbol{\beta}^c + \sigma\theta_j + \epsilon_j; \theta_j \sim N(0, 1). \tag{22.14}$$

Here, the relationship of the covariates is with each response variable rather than through the latent variable. In both models described by Eqs. (22.10) and (22.13), θ_j represents a latent construct linking the outcomes. However, the model described by Eq. (22.13) accommodates different covariate effects for each outcome, and the latent construct is conditional on these covariates. In Eq. (22.10), the covariates are the same for the binary and continuous outcomes as well as the relationship of the covariates with the outcomes. The latent construct includes the covariate effects rather than conditioning on the covariates.

In assessing quality, typically more than two quality metrics are used. Let Y_{kji} denote quality metric i measured on patient j treated by provider k. A general strategy assumes that Y^*_{kji} is an unobserved outcome that generates the observed outcome, Y_{kji}, and follows an exponential family. Then for link function l_k,

$$l_i(\mathbb{E}(Y^*_{kji} \mid \mathbf{U}_{kji}, \mathbf{X}_{kji}, \mathbf{W}_{kji}, \boldsymbol{\beta}_k, \boldsymbol{\beta}_{kj})) = \mathbf{U}^\top_{kji}\boldsymbol{\beta} + \mathbf{X}^\top_{kji}\boldsymbol{\beta}_{kj} + \mathbf{W}^\top_{kji}\boldsymbol{\beta}_k, \quad (22.15)$$

where $\boldsymbol{\beta}$ is a vector of common parameters, $\boldsymbol{\beta}_{kj}$ are within-person effects, and $\boldsymbol{\beta}_k$ are provider-specific effects. In this formulation, $\mathbf{X}_{kji} \in \mathbf{U}_{kji}$ and $\mathbf{W}_{kji} \in \mathbf{U}_{kji}$ so that $\mathbb{E}(\boldsymbol{\beta}_{kj}) = \mathbb{E}(\boldsymbol{\beta}_k) = 0$. Finally,

$$\boldsymbol{\beta}_{kj} \sim N(\mathbf{0}, \Sigma) \text{ and } \boldsymbol{\beta}_k \sim N(\mathbf{0}, \Omega). \quad (22.16)$$

Landrum et al. [90] adopted a slightly different version and used it for assessing the quality of psychiatric care across service networks within the Veterans Health Administration. For $i = 1, 2, \ldots, 8$ quality measures (4 inpatient measures and 4 outpatient measures) defined such that larger values correspond to better quality of care, the authors assumed

$$l_i(\mathbb{E}(Y^*_{kji} \mid \mathbf{U}_{kji}, \boldsymbol{\beta}_k, \phi_{kj}, \eta_{ki})) = \mathbf{U}^\top_{kji}\boldsymbol{\beta}_k + \phi_{kj} + \eta_{ki}, \quad (22.17)$$

where ϕ_{kj} accounts for within-person correlation using $\phi_{kj} \sim N(0, \tau^2)$; η_{ki} accounts for within-network correlation and models between-network heterogeneity as

$$\eta_{ki} \sim N(\lambda_{1i}\theta_{1k} + \lambda_{2i}\theta_{2k} + \cdots + \lambda_{Di}\theta_{Dk}, \psi_i^2), \quad D < 8, \quad (22.18)$$

where D is the number of latent constructs, θ_{dk} is the latent quality associated with domain d for network k, and λ_{1i} may be thought of as a factor loading. Letting $\boldsymbol{\beta}_k$ denote the D-dimensional vector of network's k quality domain, one proposed measure of a network's performance is defined by Mahalanobis squared distance, which provides a single-number summary

$$d_k^2 = (\boldsymbol{\theta}_k - \bar{\boldsymbol{\theta}})^\top \Sigma_\theta (\boldsymbol{\theta}_k - \bar{\boldsymbol{\theta}}) \quad (22.19)$$

with $\bar{\boldsymbol{\theta}} = \frac{1}{K}\sum_k(\theta_{1k}, \theta_{2k}, \ldots, \theta_{Dk})^\top$ and $\Sigma_\theta = \frac{1}{K-1}(\boldsymbol{\beta}_k - \bar{\boldsymbol{\theta}})(\boldsymbol{\beta}_k - \bar{\boldsymbol{\theta}})^\top$. Large values suggest the network k is "far" from the average across all networks. The authors identified two domains and determined the probability each network was not in the upper tail of the distribution of all distances

$$\pi_k = P(d_k^2 < \xi_{0.95} \mid \mathbf{Y}).$$

Figure 22.3 displays d_k^2 for the 22 networks and reports the probabilities π_k. Networks 7 and 15 have distances of 17.2 and 13.5, with small values of π_k, suggesting the networks are far from the other networks. Examination of the $\hat{\theta}_{1,k}$ and $\hat{\theta}_{2,k}$ for $k = 7$ and 15 indicated that network 7 had above-average quality, whereas network 15 had below-average quality.

22.4 Summary

Overall summary measures are increasingly utilized to characterize provider quality. In this chapter, we described an approach to creating composite quality measures, capitalizing on item response theory models when all metrics are discrete. Cox and Wermuth [91] discussed factorizations for modeling a continuous and a

Figure 22.3 Distance measures for 22 networks, Veterans Health Administration. Distances are defined using Eq. (22.19) for each network. The value on top of each bar is the probability the network is not in the upper tail of the distribution of all distances.

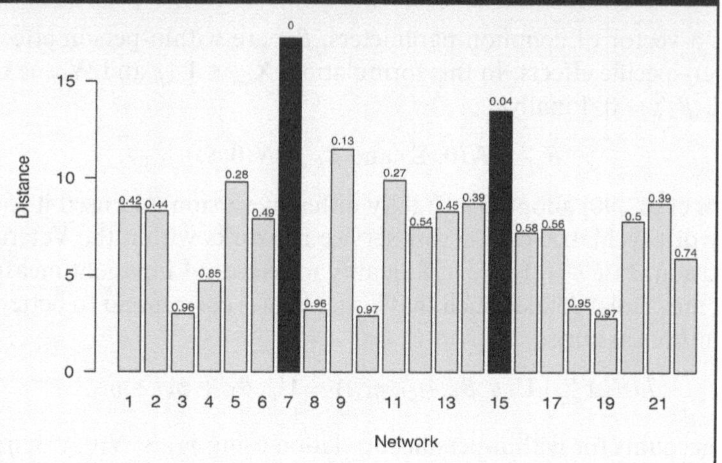

binary outcome as functions of covariates. These approaches were extended by Fitzmaurice and Laird [92] and Catalano and Ryan [93] to clustered data. Sammel et al. [89] modeled multiple outcomes assumed to be physical manifestations of a latent variable, and conditional on this latent variable, the observed outcomes follow a one-parameter exponential family model. Arminger and Küsters [94] considered each outcome as a manifestation of an underlying continuous latent variable that is normally distributed. Dunson [95] extended this approach to non-normal latent variables, clustered data, non-linear relationships between the observed outcome and the underlying variables, and multiple latent variables for each outcome type. Prentice and Zhao [96] and Zhao et al. [97] extended the GEE approach for mixtures of continuous and discrete outcomes. Papers specific to approaches for assessing healthcare quality include Normand et al. (2007) [98]; Landrum et al. (2000) [99]; Teixeira-Pinto and Normand (2008) [100]; and He et al. (2010) [86] for clustered patient aggregated data; Landrum et al. (2003) [90] for clustered mixed patient-level data; and Daniels and Normand (2006) [101] for clustered longitudinal mixed patient-level data.

CHAPTER TWENTY-THREE

Computational Approaches

Approaches to inference in a Hierarchical Generalized Linear Model (HGLM) depend on how the parameters are viewed. One approach assumes all parameters, except for the random effects, are fixed and unknown. The fixed parameters would correspond to Stages I and II regression coefficients and variance components. The other approach assumes all parameters are random. In the former case, inference focuses on the *likelihood*, while in the latter, inference focuses on the *posterior distribution* of the parameters. Recall the HGLM is

$$
\begin{aligned}
Y_{ij} \mid \boldsymbol{\theta}_i, \boldsymbol{\phi}, \mathbf{x}_{ij} &\overset{\text{indep.}}{\sim} f(Y_{ij} \mid \boldsymbol{\theta}_i, \boldsymbol{\phi}, \mathbf{x}_{ij}), \\
\boldsymbol{\theta}_i \mid \boldsymbol{\alpha}, \boldsymbol{\phi}, \mathbf{w}_i &\overset{\textit{indep.}}{\sim} g_Q(\boldsymbol{\theta}_i \mid \boldsymbol{\alpha}, \mathbf{w}_i),
\end{aligned}
$$

where Q is the number of random effects, P the number of fixed effects, and T the number of provider-specific covariates. The marginal likelihood is obtained by integrating over the random effects

$$
p(\mathbf{y_i} \mid \boldsymbol{\phi}, \boldsymbol{\alpha}, X_i, W_i) = \int_{\boldsymbol{\theta}_i} \prod_{i=1}^{I} f(\mathbf{y}_i \mid \boldsymbol{\theta}_i, \boldsymbol{\phi}, X_i) g(\boldsymbol{\theta}_i \mid \boldsymbol{\alpha}, W_i) d\boldsymbol{\theta}_i, \tag{23.1}
$$

where $\mathbf{y}_i$ is a $n_i \times 1$ vector of observations from provider i, X_i is a $n_i \times P$ design matrix of variables corresponding to fixed parameters, W_i is a $Q \times T$ design matrix of provider characteristics, and $\boldsymbol{\alpha}$ is a $T \times 1$ parameter vector.

In the Bayesian approach, inferences are based on the *posterior distribution* of the parameters given the data. Recall that prior distributions are required for all parameters, $\boldsymbol{\phi} \mid \boldsymbol{\alpha} \overset{\textit{indep.}}{\sim} h(\boldsymbol{\phi} \mid \boldsymbol{\alpha})$ and $\boldsymbol{\alpha} \sim \pi(\boldsymbol{\alpha})$. The posterior distribution is proportional to the likelihood for the data multiplied by prior distributions for the parameters

$$
p(\boldsymbol{\theta}, \boldsymbol{\phi}, \boldsymbol{\alpha} \mid \mathbf{y}, X_i, W_i) = \frac{\prod_{i=1}^{I} f(\mathbf{y}_i \mid \boldsymbol{\theta}_i, \boldsymbol{\phi}, X_i, W_i) g(\boldsymbol{\theta}_i \mid \boldsymbol{\alpha}, W_i) h(\boldsymbol{\phi} \mid \boldsymbol{\alpha}) \pi(\boldsymbol{\alpha})}{K(\mathbf{y})}. \tag{23.2}
$$

$K(\mathbf{y})$ is a normalizing constant equal to the marginal density of the data

$$
K(\mathbf{y}) = \int_{\boldsymbol{\alpha}} \int_{\boldsymbol{\phi}} \int_{\boldsymbol{\theta}_i} \prod_{i=1}^{I} f(\mathbf{y}_i \mid \boldsymbol{\theta}_i, \boldsymbol{\phi}, \boldsymbol{\alpha}, X_i, W_i) \pi^*(\boldsymbol{\theta}_i, \boldsymbol{\phi}, \boldsymbol{\alpha}) d\boldsymbol{\theta}_i d\boldsymbol{\phi} d\boldsymbol{\alpha}.
$$

Both the marginal likelihood and the Bayesian approaches require integration over many parameters, making analytical results unlikely and the computation intractable. As a result, various computational algorithms have been proposed. These approaches fall into three general categories: asymptotic approximations, numerical integration, and simulation-based integration methods. Asymptotic approximations generally do not perform well in high dimensions, and while some numerical integration approaches can handle high dimensions, they generally will not be suitable. In this chapter, we briefly review asymptotic methods and numerical integration approaches but focus mainly on iterative simulation methods because of the large number of random effects present in profiling. Simulation methods are most suitable for hierarchical modeling, and we go into greater detail on several algorithms, how to obtain a sample from the marginal or posterior distribution, and how to assess convergence when using iterative sampling. These algorithms are used in Volume 2, Chapter 24, for hypothesis testing and interval estimation.

23.1 Methods of Integration

Let $f(y)$ denote a non-negative integrable function of a random variable y, where interest lies in $\int_y f(y)dy$ or in some function of y, $g(y)$. The function, $f(y)$, could correspond to the likelihood in Eq. (23.1) that is indexed by parameters, θ, or the posterior distribution in Eq. (23.2). Henceforth, we denote $\int_y f(y)dy$ as the *target* distribution. Let $L(y)$ denote the logarithm of $f(y)$, and suppose a sample of size n is available.

23.1.1 Analytic Approximations

23.1.1.1 Normal Approximation

Classical analytic approximations based on a Normal distribution can be used to estimate $f(y)$ when the sample size, n, is large relative to the number of parameters. The idea is to expand $L(y)$ using a Taylor series about the mode, $\hat{y}$

$$L(y) \approx L(\widehat{y}) + (y - \widehat{y})\left[\frac{\partial L(y)}{\partial y}\right]_{y=\widehat{y}} + \frac{1}{2}(y - \widehat{y})^2\left[-\frac{\partial^2 L(y)}{\partial y^2}\right]_{y=\widehat{y}} + R, \quad (23.3)$$

where R is the remainder term and is of smaller order than $(y - \widehat{y})^2$. Because the mode is found by setting $\frac{\partial L(y)}{\partial y} = 0$ then $\left[\frac{\partial L(y)}{\partial y}\right]_{y-\widehat{y}} = 0$ so the second term on the right of the equal sign is 0 leaving

$$L(y) \approx L(\widehat{y}) + \frac{1}{2}(y - \widehat{y})^2\left[\frac{-\partial^2 L(y)}{\partial y^2}\right]_{y=\widehat{y}} + R.$$

Restricting to a neighborhood of $\widehat{y}$ and letting the neighborhood get smaller as the sample size $n \to \infty$, then R becomes negligible, yielding a Normal approximation to $f(y)$ defined in Box 23.1.

Box 23.1 Normal approximation to $f(y)$

$$y \dot{\sim} N\left(\widehat{y}, \left\{\left[\frac{-\partial^2 L(y)}{\partial y^2}\right]_{y=\widehat{y}}\right\}^{-1}\right). \quad (23.4)$$

Box 23.2 Laplace approximation to $\int_y f(y)dy$

$$\int_y f(y)dy \approx \exp L(\widehat{y})\sqrt{2\pi}\sigma \exp L(\widehat{y}). \quad (23.6)$$

In general, $I(\hat{y}) = \left\{\left[\frac{-\partial^2 L(y)}{\partial y^2}\right]_{y=\widehat{y}}\right\}^{-1}$, the observed Fisher Information, and $\widehat{y}$ are not difficult to compute. The mode, which requires maximization, is easier to find than the mean, which requires integration. If no closed-form expression exists, then a Newton–Raphson algorithm (described below) can be applied to find the mode. Inferences, such as hypothesis testing and confidence interval construction, are based on assuming y arises from a Normal distribution described in Box 23.1.

23.1.1.2 Laplace Approximation

A different approximation is based on Laplace's method suggested by Tierney and Kadane [102], in which a Taylor series expansion of $\int_y f(y)dy$ about its mode, $\widehat{y}$, is used rather than an expansion of $L(y)$. The authors include a third term in Eq. (23.3) expansion,

$$L(y) \approx L(\widehat{y}) + \frac{1}{2}(y-\widehat{y})^2\left[-\frac{\partial^2 L(y)}{\partial y^2}\right]_{y=\widehat{y}} + \frac{1}{3!}(y-\widehat{y})^3\left[-\frac{\partial^3 L(y)}{\partial y^3}\right]_{y=\widehat{y}} + R, \quad (23.5)$$

where the linear term is removed because $y = \widehat{y}$. Now

$$\int_y f(y)dy = \int_Y \exp L(y)dy \approx \exp L(\widehat{y}) \int_y \exp\frac{(y-\widehat{y})^2}{2\sigma^2} \underbrace{\int_y \exp\frac{(y-\widehat{y})^3}{3!\delta^2}dy}_{\text{A}},$$

where $\sigma^2 = \left\{\left[\frac{-\partial^2 L(y)}{\partial y^2}\right]_{y=\widehat{y}}\right\}^{-1}$ and $\delta^2 = \left\{\left[\frac{-\partial^3 L(y)}{\partial y^3}\right]_{y=\widehat{y}}\right\}^{-1}$. Next, expand the term A about $\widehat{y}$ which yields

$$\begin{aligned}\int_y f(y)dy &= \int_y \exp L(y)dy \\ &\approx \exp L(\widehat{y}) \int_y \exp\frac{(y-\widehat{y})^2}{2\sigma^2}\left[1 + \frac{(y-\widehat{y})^3}{3!\delta^2} + \frac{(y-\widehat{y})^6}{2(3!)^2\delta^4} + R\right]dy.\end{aligned}$$

A first-order approximation to $\int_y f(y)$ ignores the last 3 terms, yielding the Laplace approximation to the integral in Box 23.2.

Importantly, functions of y can be determined through a similar expansion. For instance, $\mathbb{E}(g(y))$ can be approximated by replacing $L(y)$ with $L^*(y) = \log g(y) + L(y)$ in Eq. (23.5). Like the Normal approximation, these results are valid only asymptotically, requiring $f(y)$ to be peaked about $\widehat{y}$.

Both the Laplace and Normal asymptotic approximations are computationally quick because they do not rely on an iterative algorithm. The approaches place numerical integration with numerical differentiation, which is often easier and more stable. The accuracy of approximation does depend on the parameterization utilized, such as y versus $\log(y)$. For moderate to high dimensions, dimensions $\geqslant 10$, neither method will be of sufficient accuracy; numerical computation of the associated matrices (derivatives) will be prohibitively difficult.

23.1.2 Numerical Integration

Numerical integration algorithms are designed to provide close approximations to the likelihood or posterior distribution without resorting to Normal approximations.

23.1.2.1 Trapezoidal Rule

The trapezoidal rule uses a grid of points $\{y^0, y^1, \ldots, y^n\}$ that cover the region over which $f(y)$ is appreciably non-zero. The areas of the trapezoids whose vertices are

$$(y^j, 0),\ (y^{j+1}, 0),\ (y^{j+1}, f(y^{j+1})),\ (y^j, f(y^j))$$

are summed. Therefore,

$$\int_y f(y)dy \approx \sum_{j=0}^{n-1} \left[(y^{j+1} - y^j) \min\left(f(y^j), f(y^{j+1})\right) + \frac{1}{2}(y^{j+1} - y^j) \left| f(y^{j+1}) - f(y^j) \right| \right].$$

If $f(y)$ has very heavy tails, then it may be difficult to determine the correct range $\left[y^0, y^n\right]$ required to get good results. The sensitivity of the results can be assessed by using a variety of grids. Numerical integration can sometimes be used in multiparameter problems if integration of all dimensions except one can be achieved analytically. Suppose $\mathbf{y} = (y_1, y_2, \ldots, y_I)$ and $f(y)$ can be written as

$$f(\mathbf{y}) = f(y_2, y_3, \ldots, y_I \mid y_1) f(y_1),$$

where $f(y_2, y_3, \ldots, y_I \mid y_1)$ is tractable. In this case, only a one-dimensional numerical integration over y_1 is required. However, in higher-dimension problems, numerical integration becomes impractical (e.g., if >3 dimensions).

23.1.2.2 Gaussian–Hermite Quadrature

Gaussian (or Gauss–Hermite) quadrature [103] approximates $\int_y f(y)dy$, as a weighted sum of orthogonal polynomials, assuming $f(y)$ is well approximated by the *product* of a multivariate Normal and a polynomial. Consider the univariate setting and let $h(y)$ be approximately polynomial and define

Box 23.3 Gaussian–Hermite quadrature algorithm

$$\int_{-\infty}^{\infty} s(y)dy \approx \sum_{i=1}^{n} m_i g(z_i) \tag{23.7}$$

where $m_i = w_i \exp(y_i^2)\sqrt{2}\sigma$ and $z_i = \mu + \sqrt{2}\sigma y_i$. Tables containing values for y_i, w_i, and $w_i \exp(y_i^2)$ exist.

Box 23.4 Newton–Raphson algorithm

Generate an initial guess, $y^{(0)}$.

1. At iteration i determine

$$y^{(i+1)} = y^{(i)} + \left(-\frac{\partial^2 L(y)}{\partial y^2}\Big|_{y^{(i)}} \right)^{-1} \left[\frac{\partial L(y)}{\partial y}\Big|_{y^{(i)}} \right]. \tag{23.8}$$

2. If $y^{(i+1)} - y^{(i)}$ is sufficiently small, STOP. Otherwise, go back to Step 1 setting i to $i+1$.

$$s(y) = \frac{h(y)}{\sqrt{2\pi}\sigma} \exp\left\{ -\frac{1}{2}\left(\frac{y-\mu}{\sigma} \right)^2 \right\}.$$

Then adaptive quadrature evaluated at n points is provided in Box 23.3.

The error of the approximation if $h(y)$ is approximately a polynomial function.[1] This approach has been found to work well up to 8 dimensions.

23.1.2.3 Newton–Raphson Algorithm

We return to the Taylor series expansion of $L(y)$ about some point, $y^{(i)}$ close to the mode

$$L(y) \approx L(y^{(i)}) + (y - y^{(i)}) \left[\frac{\partial L(y)}{\partial y} \right]_{y=y^{(i)}} + \frac{1}{2}(y - y^{(i)})^2 \left[-\frac{\partial^2 L(y)}{\partial y^2} \right]_{y=y^{(i)}} + R.$$

One can show that

$$y^{(i+1)} = y^{(i)} + \left(-\frac{\partial^2 L(y)}{\partial y^2}\Big|_{y^{(i)}} \right)^{-1} \left[\frac{\partial L(y)}{\partial y}\Big|_{y^{(i)}} \right]$$

by determining the stationary point in the series expansion. This leads to the algorithm in Box 23.4.

Only one iteration is required if the log-likelihood is quadratic. If the log-likelihood is concave and unimodal, the sequence of iterations converges to the mode.

[1] A polynomial function of t of order n is defined as $P(t) = a_0 + a_1 t + a_2 t^2 + \cdots a_n t^n$ where a_i is a constant and $a_n \neq 0$.

23.1.3 Non-iterative Simulation-Based Integration Methods

23.1.3.1 Direct Sampling

Suppose the goal is to compute $E(g(y))$ for some function g where y has density $f(y)$. By definition,

$$\gamma = \mathbb{E}(g(y)) = \int_y g(y)f(y)dy.$$

If $y^1, y^2, \ldots, y^N$ are i.i.d. samples drawn from $f(y)$, then the Monte Carlo approximation to γ is

$$\widehat{\gamma} = \frac{1}{N}\sum_{j=1}^{N} g(y^j).$$

The estimator, $\hat{\gamma}$, converges to $\mathbb{E}(g(y))$ with probability one as $N \to \infty$ by the strong law of large numbers. The key condition is the ability to directly sample from $f(y)$, for example, $f(y)$ is known. Computation of the expectation requires a sample of size N from $f(y)$ and as N increases, the quality of the approximation increases. Moreover, $\mathrm{Var}(\widehat{\gamma}) = \frac{1}{N}\mathrm{Var}(g(y))$ because the y^i's are drawn independently. The $\mathrm{Var}(g(y))$ can be estimated by the sample variance of $g(y)$,

$$\mathrm{Var}(\widehat{\gamma}) = \frac{1}{N(N-1)}\sum_{j=1}^{N}\left(g(y^j) - \widehat{\gamma}\right)^2.$$

A distinct advantage of Monte Carlo integration is the ease of estimating quantities other than the mean. For example, suppose we are interested in estimating $p = P(a < g(y) < b)$. Then

$$\widehat{p} = \frac{1}{N}\sum_{i=1}^{N} I(g(y^i) \in (a,b)) \text{ and } V(\widehat{p}) = \frac{\widehat{p}(1-\widehat{p})}{N},$$

where $I(g(y^i) \in (a,b)) = 1$ if $g(y^i) \in (a,b)$ and 0 otherwise. An estimate of the entire distribution could also be obtained by constructing a histogram of the sampled y^j's.

23.1.3.2 Indirect Methods

The more common situation is one for which sampling directly from $f(y)$ is not possible. In this setting, several noniterative approaches are available.

Importance Sampling. This strategy samples from a known distribution and then weights the draw by how close the known density evaluated at the draw is to the target density at the draw [104]. Suppose interest lies in $E(g(y))$ for some function g.

$$\mathbb{E}(g(y)) = \int_y g(y)f(y)dy = \int_y g(y)\frac{f(y)}{h(y)}h(y)dy,$$

where $h(y)$ is some density from which it is easy to sample (e.g., multivariate Student t distribution). The function $h(y)$ is called the *importance function.* Using Monte Carlo simulation, $\mathbb{E}(g(y))$ can be approximated by

Box 23.5 Rejection/Acceptance sampling algorithm

1. Generate $y^j \sim h(y)$.
2. Generate $u^j \sim \text{Uniform}(0, 1)$.
3. If $Mu^j h(y^j) < f(y^j)$ then accept y^j, otherwise reject y^j.
4. Go back to Step (1) until the desired sample is obtained $\{y^j,\ j = 1, 2, \ldots, N\}$. The elements of this set will be random variables sampled from $f(y)$.

$$\mathbb{E}(g(y)) \approx \frac{1}{N} \sum_{j=1}^{N} g(y^j) \frac{f(y^j)}{h(y^j)}.$$

If $h(y)$ is a good approximation to $f(y)$, then the weights, $f(y)/h(y)$, will be approximately equal. When $h(y)$ is a poor approximation, then many of the weights will be close to zero so that few y^j's will dominate the sums, resulting in an inaccurate approximation.

Rejection/Acceptance Sampling. This approach is very general and commonly used to generate random variables (see Devroye [105] for a summary). Rather than approximating $f(y)$, the idea is to blanket $f(y)$. Suppose there exists an identifiable constant M and smooth density $h(y)$ such that

$$f(y) < Mh(y) \qquad \forall y.$$

The density $h(y)$ is called the envelope function or a majorizing function. If such a function exists, then the algorithm described in Box 23.5 is used.

The goal is to have M as small as possible so as not to waste samples. If k denotes the number of iterations required to get one acceptable candidate y^j, then

$$P(k = i) = (1 - P)^{i-1} P$$

where P is the probability of acceptance, $\frac{\int_y f(y)dy}{M}$. Because $\mathbb{E}(k) = P^{-1} = \frac{M}{\int_y f(y)dy}$, minimizing M is desirable. The envelope density, $h(y)$, should be similar to $f(y)$ but have heavier tails and sharper peaks to cover the entire domain.

Importance sampling and rejection/acceptance sampling are non-iterative methods: A sample of size N is drawn, and then you stop. One simply requires N to be sufficiently large. However, in many problems, particularly high dimensional problems, it may be quite difficult to find an importance sampling density (or an envelope function), which will be an acceptably accurate approximation to $f(y)$ and from which it will be easy to sample. Consequently, iterative Monte Carlo methods have been proposed, and these approaches are described next.

23.1.4 Iterative Simulation-Based Integration Methods

Markov Chain Monte Carlo (MCMC) refers to a set of iterative algorithms used to sample from a probability distribution. The algorithm yields a *Markov chain* that evolves to the target distribution. A Markov chain is a sequence of random variables that evolve. We focus on an algorithm referred to as the *Gibbs sampler*, which is a specific case of the more general *Metropolis–Hastings* algorithm.

23.1.4.1 The Gibbs Sampler

Suppose we have a collection of I random variables denoted by $\mathbf{Y} = (y_1, \ldots, y_I)$. We assume that the *full conditional distributions*

$$\{f(y_i \mid y_j, \ j \neq i), \ i = 1, \ldots, I\}$$

are available for sampling; that is, the samples may be generated by some method. Thus, the one-dimensional conditional distributions $[y_i \mid y_j, \ j \neq i]$, $i = 1, \ldots, I$ need not have a closed form, although they need to be known up to a normalizing constant. Under mild conditions [106], the one-dimensional conditional distributions uniquely determine the full joint distribution of $\mathbf{Y}$ and hence all marginal distributions $[y_i]$, $i = 1, \ldots, I$. Without loss of generality, let $[Y_1 \mid Y_2]$ denote the conditional distribution of Y_1 given Y_2. Box 23.6 describes an algorithm, denoted *Gibbs sampling* [107], to determine the joint distribution.

For the Gibbs sampling algorithm outlined above, $(y_1^{(t)}, \ldots, y_I^{(t)}) \xrightarrow{d} [y_1, \ldots, y_I]$ as $t \to \infty$ and the convergence is exponential in t. For proofs of these theorems, see Geman and Geman [108] and Schervish and Carlin [109]. Gelfand and Smith [110] exposed this algorithm to statisticians in the context of Bayesian inference. The algorithm shows that sampling from $f(\mathbf{Y})$ requires draws from each of the univariate conditional distributions $f(Y_i \mid \mathbf{Y}_{-i})$, where $\mathbf{Y}_{-i} = (y_1, \ldots, y_{i-1}, yx_{i+1}, \ldots y_I)$. When t is sufficiently large, then a marginal density estimate of y_i is given by

$$\widehat{f}(y_i \mid \mathbf{y}_{-i}) = \frac{1}{m-t} \sum_{t=t+1}^{m} f(y_i \mid y_1^{(t)}, y_{i-1}^{(t)}, y_{i+1}^{(t)}, \ldots, y_I^{(t)}).$$

The sequence $\mathbf{y}^{(1)}, \mathbf{y}^{(2)}, \ldots, \mathbf{y}^{(t)}$ is called the *burn-in*.

Example: Normal Data (Box 23.7). Let $y \overset{\text{iid}}{\sim} N(\mu, \sigma^2)$ with a total of $n = 10$ observations. Suppose $y = 78, 66, 65, 63, 60, 60, 58, 56, 52, 50$ so that $\bar{y} = 60.8$ and $s^2 = 63.5$. Assume the prior distribution for $\pi(\mu, \sigma^2) \ \propto \ \sigma^{-2}$. To implement the Gibbs sampler, the full conditional distributions are required. In this example, the full conditionals are

$$\mu \mid \mathbf{y}, \sigma^2 \sim N\left(\bar{y}, \frac{\sigma^2}{n}\right) \quad \text{and} \quad \sigma^2 \mid \mathbf{y}, \mu \sim \left\{\sum_{1}^{n} (y_i - \mu)^2\right\} \chi_n^{-2}.$$

Box 23.6 Gibbs Sampling algorithm

0) Suppose we have a set of arbitrary starting values $\{y_1^{(0)}, \ldots, y_I^{(0)}\}$.
1) Draw $y_1^{(1)}$ from $[y_1 \mid y_2^{(0)}, \ldots, y_I^{(0)}]$
2) Draw $y_2^{(1)}$ from $[y_2 \mid y_1^{(1)}, y_3^{(0)}, \ldots, y_I^{(0)}]$

⋮

I) Draw $y_I^{(1)}$ from $[y_I \mid y_1^{(1)}, \ldots, y_{I-1}^{(1)}]$

This completes one iteration of the Gibbs sampler so that after iteration 1, one draw of $\mathbf{y}^{(1)} = (y_1^{(1)}, \ldots, y_I^{(1)})$ is obtained. After t such iterations, a single draw of $\mathbf{y}^t$ defined by $(y_1^{(t)}, \ldots, y_I^{(t)})$ is obtained. The series of draws, $\mathbf{y}^{(1)}, \mathbf{y}^{(2)}, \ldots, \mathbf{y}^{(t)}$ is called a *chain*.

Box 23.7 Gibbs Sampling algorithm for Normal Model

0) Starting values $\{\mu^{(0)} = 60.8, \sigma^{2(0)} = 63.5\}$.
1) Draw $\mu^{(1)}$ from $N\left(\mu^{(0)}, \sigma^{2(0)}\right)$
2) Draw $\sigma^{2(1)}$ from χ_{10}^{-2} and multiply by $\left\{\sum_1^{10}(y_i - \mu^{(1)})^2\right\}$

This completes one iteration of the Gibbs sampler. After t (t large), draw S more samples and use these to summarize means, variances, and other features of the distribution.

Box 23.8 Metropolis algorithm

1. Draw $v \sim q(\cdot, y)$, where $y = y^{(t-1)}$, the current state of the Metropolis algorithm.
2. Compute the odds ratio

$$r = \frac{p(v)}{p(y)}$$

3. If $r \geqslant 1$, set $y^{(t)} = v$ (acceptance)
4. If $r < 1$, set

$$y^{(t)} = \begin{cases} v & \text{with probability } r \\ y & \text{with probability } 1 - r \end{cases}$$

(rejection)

In this simple case, the marginal posterior distributions of the parameters are known exactly, specifically,

$$\sigma^2 \mid \mathbf{y} \sim (n-1)s^2\chi_{n-1}^{-2} \quad \text{and} \quad \mu \mid \mathbf{y} \sim t_{n-1}\left(\bar{y}, \frac{(n-1)s^2}{n}\right).$$

The starting values, while permitted to be arbitrary, should be wisely selected. In the example above, the observed mean and variance of the sample data are used. This is permitted, as these values are used only as starting values and do not influence the final inferences.

23.1.4.2 Metropolis–Hastings Algorithm

The Metropolis algorithm is a general MCMC method proposed by Metropolis et al. [111] and introduced to statistical problems by Hastings [112]. Suppose we wish to sample from the joint distribution $[y_1, \ldots, y_k] = [y]$, where $y = (y_1, \ldots, y_k)$. Denote the density of y by $p(y)$. Let $q(v, y)$ be a density in y such that $q(y, v) = q(v, y)$. The function q is called a *candidate* or *proposal* density. Box 23.8 describes how values are sampled.

For the Metropolis algorithm, under mild conditions, $[y^{(t)}] \rightarrow [y]$ as $t \rightarrow \infty$. For continuous random variables, the most convenient choice for q is a $N(y^{(t-1)}, \tilde{\Sigma})$, where $\tilde{\Sigma}$ can be taken as

$$\tilde{\Sigma} = -\left[\frac{\partial^2 \log[f(y)]}{\partial y\, \partial y'}\right]^{-1}\Bigg|_{y=y^{(t-1)}}.$$

Box 23.9 Metropolis–Hastings algorithm

1. Draw $v \sim q(\cdot, y)$, where $y = y^{(t-1)}$, the current state of the Metropolis algorithm.
2. Compute the odds ratio

$$r = \frac{p(v)\, q(y, v)}{p(y)\, q(v, y)}$$

3. If $r \geqslant 1$, set $y^{(t)} = v$ (acceptance)
4. If $r < 1$, set

$$y^{(t)} = \begin{cases} v & \text{with probability } r \\ y & \text{with probability } 1 - r \end{cases}$$

(rejection)

This choice of q is easily sampled and clearly symmetric in v and $y^{(t-1)}$.

A simple but important generalization of the Metropolis algorithm was provided by Hastings [112] that resulted in eliminating the requirement that $q(y, v)$ be symmetric. and redefined the odds ratio to yield a different algorithm (Box 23.9),

With this modification, it can be shown that this algorithm converges to the required "target" distribution for any candidate density q. Chib and Greenberg [113] give an excellent discussion of the Metropolis–Hastings algorithms and discuss choices of $q(y, v)$.

The Metropolis–Hastings algorithm involves updating an entire vector of parameters each time. Gibbs sampling is a simpler version of the Metropolis–Hastings algorithm. It uses the conditional distribution as the proposal distribution; hence, it always accepts each draw.

23.1.4.3 Convergence

How does one determine if t is sufficiently large? An MCMC algorithm has converged at iteration t if its output can be safely thought of as coming from the target distribution of the Markov chain for all $s > t$. Sometimes there may be convergence difficulty, mostly due to model over-parameterization, making the parameters non-identifiable. Consider finding the distribution of θ_1, where the likelihood is defined by

$$x_i \mid \theta_1, \theta_2 \overset{i.i.d.}{\sim} N(\theta_1 + \theta_2, 1)\,,$$

$i = 1, \ldots, n$. Suppose we adopt a Bayesian approach and take $\pi(\theta_1, \theta_2) \propto 1$, which is not a proper prior distribution. In this example, only the sum of the two parameters is identified by the data; the marginal distributions are not identifiable. A naive application of the Gibbs sampler in this setting would not reveal this problem.

Additionally, models that are over-parameterized typically lead to high posterior correlations among the parameters. These correlations are referred to as *cross-correlations*. High cross-correlations will dramatically affect the movement of the Gibbs sampler through the parameter space. Even if the parameters are identifiable, high cross-correlations and high auto-correlations can lead to slow convergence. One remedy suggested for reducing high correlations among parameters

Box 23.10 Scale reduction factor for convergence

1. Run a small number (m) of parallel chains with different starting points.
2. These chains must be initially **overdispersed** to the true posterior.
3. Running the m chains for $2N$ iterations each, check whether the *variation within the chains* for a given parameter of interest, say λ, approximately equals the *total variation across* chains during the latter N iterations.
4. Calculate the estimated *scale reduction factor*,

$$\sqrt{\widehat{R}} = \sqrt{\left(\frac{N-1}{N} + \frac{m+1}{mN}\frac{B}{W}\right)\left(\frac{df}{df-2}\right)},$$

   where B/N is the variance between the means from the m parallel chains, W is the average of the m within-chain variances, and df is the degrees of freedom of an approximating t density to the posterior distribution.
5. The goal is to have $\widehat{R} = 1$.

is reparameterization. Gelfand et al. [114] discuss a class of transformations called *hierarchical centering*, which is quite useful for hierarchical models. In general, finding appropriate reparameterizations is difficult.

Diagnostic statistics that assess convergence have been developed. These convergence diagnostics have a wide range of characteristics. Most diagnostics address the issue of bias, that is, the distance of the estimated quantities of interest at a particular iteration from their true values under the target distribution. A few also consider the variance, or the precision of the draws. Some diagnostics are quantitative, producing a single-number summary, while others are qualitative, summarized by a graph or other display. Some diagnostics may be implemented using only a single MCMC chain, while others require a small number of parallel chains created by initiating each chain from different starting values. Finally, some diagnostics consider only univariate quantities, while others attempt to diagnose convergence of the full joint distribution.

Perhaps the single most popular approach is due to Gelman and Rubin [115], based on a scalar summary who demonstrated that $\sqrt{\widehat{R}} \to 1$ as $N \to \infty$ (see Box 23.10). Thus, values of $\sqrt{\widehat{R}}$ close to 1 suggest good convergence. This approach has been criticized for several reasons. First, it is a univariate diagnostic. It must be applied to each parameter. Thus, if $\mathbf{y} = (y_1, \ldots, y_I)$, one needs to compute $\sqrt{\widehat{R}_{y_j}}$, $j = 1, \ldots, I$. Second, the approach focuses solely on the bias component of convergence, providing no information as to the accuracy of the resulting estimates. Third, the method relies heavily on the user's ability to find a starting distribution that is over-dispersed to the target distribution of y, a condition that cannot be determined without knowledge of the target distribution.

Geyer [116] recommends a different approach, wherein a single chain is used, and the focus is not on the bias but on the variance of the resulting estimates. For example, letting $\widehat{y}_N = \frac{1}{N}\sum_{t=1}^{N} y^{(t)}$, by the central limit theorem,

$$\sqrt{N}\,(\widehat{y}_N - y) \xrightarrow{d} N(0, \sigma^2)\,,$$

where σ^2 can be estimated by

$$\widehat{\sigma}_N^2 = \sum_{t=-\infty}^{\infty} w_N(t)\, \widehat{\gamma}_{N,t}.$$

Here, $w_N(t)$ is a weight function called a lag window, and $\widehat{\gamma}_{N,t}$ is an estimate of the lag t autocovariance function, namely

$$\widehat{\gamma}_{N,t} = \frac{1}{N} \sum_{i=1}^{N-t} \left(y^{(i)} - \widehat{y}_N\right) \left(y^{(i+t)} - \widehat{y}_N\right).$$

The lag window satisfies $0 \leqslant w_N(t) \leqslant 1$ and is used to downweight the large-lag terms. An approximate 95% confidence interval for $\mathbb{E}(y)$ is thus obtainable as

$$\widehat{y}_N \pm 1.96 \frac{\widehat{\sigma}_N}{\sqrt{N}} .$$

The above formulae assume no discarding of early samples (i.e., no burn-in). Geyer argues that less than 1% of the run will normally be a sufficient burn-in period whenever the run is long enough to give much precision.[2]

Geyer's approach addresses the variance goal and avoids parallel chains or any notion of "initial overdispersion." However, it does not generalize well beyond moments, such as quantiles or density estimates for y, and it does not assess bias.

A computationally simpler method of estimating $\text{Var}(\hat{y}_N)$ is through *batching*. Suppose a single long run of length $N = mk$ is conducted. Divide the run into m successive batches of length k with batch means $B_1, \ldots, B_m$. We have

$$\hat{y}_N = \bar{B} = \frac{1}{m} \sum_{i=1}^{m} B_i \quad \text{with} \quad \widehat{V} \equiv \widehat{\text{Var}}(\hat{y}_N) = \frac{1}{m(m-1)} \sum_{i=1}^{m} (B_i - \hat{y}_N)^2,$$

provided that k is large enough so that the correlation between batches is negligible, and m is large enough to reliably estimate $\text{Var}(B_i)$ The confidence interval for $\mathbb{E}(y)$ is then given by

$$\widehat{y}_N \pm t_{(m-1,.025)} \sqrt{\widehat{V}},$$

where $t_{(m-1,.025)}$ is the upper 0.025 point of a t distribution with $m-1$ degrees of freedom.

Another solution to estimating $\text{Var}(\widehat{y}_N)$ would be to simply use the sample variance of the kth iteration output from m independent parallel chains. However, this approach is wasteful, discarding $\frac{k-1}{k}$ of the samples. Raftery and Lewis [117] developed a diagnostic aimed at accurately estimating posterior quantiles.

Cowles and Carlin [118] provide a nice overview of several convergence diagnostic statistics. In summary:

1. Run a few (3–5) parallel chains, with starting points drawn from a distribution believed to be overdispersed to the stationary distribution (say, covering $\pm$ 3 prior standard deviations from the prior mean).

[2] Recall that Gelman and Rubin discard the first 50% of each chain.

2. Visually inspect these chains by overlaying their sampled values on a common graph for each parameter, or, for very high-dimensional models, a representative subset of the parameters.
3. Annotate each graph with the Gelman and Rubin [115] statistic and lag 1 autocorrelations. Large Gelman and Rubin (1992) statistics may arise from either slow mixing or multimodality.
4. Investigate cross-correlations among parameters suspected of being nearly non-identifiable.

An area closely related to convergence diagnosis is that of convergence acceleration. Reparameterizations can often improve a model's correlation structure and hence accelerate convergence. The closer the correlations are to 0, the faster the convergence.

23.1.4.4 Obtaining a Sample of Size *s* from the Distribution

Let $y_i^{(j)}$ denote the *j*th *iterate* from the *i*th *chain*, and assume convergence after *t* iterations (see Table (23.1) for a schematic of the draws). The initial values, $y_i^{(0)}$, differ across the chains. Three possible sampling schemes of the draws can be used to obtain a sample of size s from the posterior distribution.

Independent Sample

Use *s* chains: $\left\{y_1^{(t+1)}, y_2^{(t+1)}, \ldots, y_s^{(t+1)}\right\}$. If the chains are initialized independently, the sample will consist of independent values from the posterior distribution. This option requires the generation of $s(t+1)$ values from the chains.

Single Chain

Use a single chain, *i*: $\left\{y_i^{(t+1)}, y_i^{(t+2)}, \ldots, y_i^{(t+s)}\right\}$. The sample elements are no longer independent because of chain dependence, and the samples should be checked to ensure the autocorrelation is not too high. This option requires $t+s$ generations from the chain, substantially less than the independent sampling approach.

Table 23.1 Draws of random variables, *y*, using the Gibbs sampler.

	Iterations						
Chain	1	2	$\cdots$	t	$t+1$	$\cdots$	$t+s$
1	$y_1^{(0)}$	$y_1^{(1)}$	$\cdots$	$y_1^{(t)}$	$y_1^{(t+1)}$	$\cdots$	$y_1^{(t+s)}$
2	$y_2^{(0)}$	$y_2^{(1)}$	$\cdots$	$y_2^{(t)}$	$y_2^{(t+1)}$	$\cdots$	$y_2^{(t+s)}$
$\vdots$	$\vdots$	$\vdots$	$\vdots$	$\vdots$	$\vdots$	$\vdots$	$\vdots$
s	$y_s^{(0)}$	$y_s^{(1)}$	$\cdots$	$y_s^{tm)}$	$y_s^{(t+1)}$	$\cdots$	$y_s^{(t+s)}$

Quasi-Independent
Use a single chain i, $\left\{y_i^{(t+k)}, y_i^{(t+2k)}, \ldots, y_i^{(t+sk)}\right\}$ for $0 < k < t$. This option requires $t + ks$ generations from the chain. However, estimation (of functions of y) is less precise than retaining all chain values.

23.1.5 Variational Bayes

Another approach commonly adopted in the Bayesian setting is to approximate the (posterior) distribution by solving a constrained minimization problem. The idea is to use a tractable distribution, $q(y)$, to approximate the target distribution $f(y)$. The approach uses the Kullback–Leibler divergence from $q(y)$ to $f(y)$. The approximation to $f(y)$ is obtained by

$$q* = \arg\min_{q \in \mathcal{Q}} \left\{ KL(y) = \int q(y) \log \frac{q(y)}{f(y)} dy \right\}. \tag{23.9}$$

$KL(y) = 0$ if and only if $q(y) = f(y)$. For a comprehensive review of these methods, see Nakajima et al. (2019) [119].

23.2 Summary

A comprehensive literature exists on numerical and Monte Carlo methods for integration. Interested readers should see Geweke (1995) [120] and references therein. We began with a description of approximations based on a Taylor series expansion of the log-likelihood function and then discussed some noniterative numerical methods. Because most of these methods are not suitable in high dimensions, which is the norm for assessing healthcare providers, we focused on Markov Chain Monte Carlo sampling. These methods are suitable in high-dimensional settings and provide a sample of draws from the target distribution. These draws are then used for inferences, which is the subject of the next chapter.

CHAPTER TWENTY-FOUR

Inference for Hierarchical Generalized Linear Models

The prior chapter described computational strategies for integrating over distributions that are required for determining joint and marginal distributions. Approaches to making inferences, such as hypothesis testing or constructing confidence intervals, are discussed in this chapter using frequentist and Bayesian approaches. Both approaches utilize the likelihood function of the observed data. A maximum likelihood estimator (MLE) for a parameter, $\boldsymbol{\beta}$, is the value of $\boldsymbol{\beta}$ that maximizes the likelihood or the log-likelihood. When the likelihood is differentiable and unimodal, the MLE is obtained by differentiating the log-likelihood to $\boldsymbol{\beta}$, setting the resulting derivative equations to 0, and solving for $\boldsymbol{\beta}$. However, the *likelihood principle* states that the likelihood function contains all the information in the observed data about *fixed* parameters and thus provides no basis for making inferences about the *random effects*. For this reason, *extended maximum likelihood* was proposed as a framework for estimating both the fixed and random parameters. In this approach, constraints on the parameters characterizing the random effects distribution are imposed.

Empirical Bayes and fully Bayesian approaches also rely on the likelihood function. A fully Bayesian approach updates the likelihood of the parameters with prior information. No constraints on the distribution of the random effects are required. However, prior distributions for all model parameters must be specified. Empirical Bayes approaches use the data to estimate the parameters of the random effects distributions and plug these estimates into MLEs.

Other inferential approaches are available for clustered data. For instance, quasi-likelihood approaches only make assumptions about the first two moments of the distribution for the outcomes, avoiding the need to completely specify the distribution. For clustered data, the second moment amounts to describing a covariance structure that reflects the dependence induced by within-cluster correlation. While quasi-likelihood approaches accommodate clustered data, they treat the between-cluster covariance parameters as nuisance parameters. Earlier chapters described the key role played by both the between-provider covariance parameters and the random effects in assessing healthcare providers. For this reason, quasi-likelihood approaches are not discussed further. Readers should see Wedderburn (1974) [121] and references therein for a complete treatment of quasi-likelihood approaches.

We begin this chapter by briefly describing how inferences may be obtained from frequentist and Bayesian approaches. Methods for inferences in the HLM are then discussed. To link to the vast literature on generalized linear mixed models (GLLM), we recast the HLM as a GLLM. Inferences for HGLMs using extended likelihood and Bayesian approaches are next discussed. Several examples are discussed.

24.1 Approaches to Inference

24.1.1 Maximum Likelihood

The likelihood principle states that evidence from an experiment depends on the data only through the likelihood. When the log likelihood function is approximately quadratic, inference for fixed parameters, denoted θ, proceeds by computing the first two derivatives of the log likelihood, $l(\theta)$. The *score function* is the derivative of the log likelihood function,

$$S(\theta) = \frac{\partial l(\theta)}{\partial \theta}.$$

The maximum likelihood estimator (MLE), $\widehat{\theta}$, is the solution to the score equation, $S(\theta) = 0$. The negative of the expected *Fisher Information*

$$I(\theta) = -E\left(\frac{\partial^2 l(\theta)}{\partial \theta^2}\right)$$

measures the curvature of the log likelihood at the maximum. Large values of $I(\theta)$ suggest the log likelihood is peaked, so that there is more certainty about the location of the maximum. Assuming some regularity conditions, the law of large numbers, and the central limit theorem, if θ is the true value, then the MLE

$$\widehat{\theta} \sim N(\theta, I^{-1}(\widehat{\theta})). \tag{24.1}$$

If θ has length greater than 1, then $I(\widehat{\theta})$[1] is a matrix, and the variance for the ith component of $\widehat{\theta}$ is the i-i element of $I(\widehat{\theta})$. Confidence intervals can be constructed using the Normal distribution. Hypothesis tests are conducted using the Wald statistic with a standard Normal null distribution. For instance, a test of $H_0 : \theta = \theta_0$ uses the test statistic

$$z = \frac{\widehat{\theta} - \theta_0}{se(\widehat{\theta})}.$$

Because the log-likelihood for a hierarchical model is often intractable, the computation strategies discussed in Volume 2, Chapter 23, "Computational Approaches," are adopted.

24.1.2 Bayesian Inference

The two ingredients for the Bayesian approach are the likelihood, generally referred to as the sample distribution of the observed data, $f(y \mid \theta)$, and a prior distribution

[1] $I(\widehat{\theta})$ is the *observed Fisher Information* and used in Volume 2, Chapter 23, "Computational Approaches."

for the parameters, $\pi(\theta)$. Inference for the parameters contained in θ is based on the posterior distribution of the parameters given the observed data obtained using Bayes formula,

$$p(\theta \mid y) = \frac{f(y \mid \theta)\pi(\theta)}{\int_\theta f(y \mid \theta)\pi(\theta)d\theta} = \frac{f(y \mid \theta)\pi(\theta)}{m(y)}.$$

The term $m(y)$ is the marginal distribution of y obtained by integrating over the parameter space and plays a role in empirical Bayes inference.[2] There is no unique way of choosing a prior distribution, and the choice of the prior distribution can impact the conclusions drawn if the number of observations is small. In hierarchical models, prior distributions are required at all levels of the hierarchy, and, generally, the prior distribution for the variance components at higher stages of the hierarchy can be influential.

Subjective prior distributions incorporate specific information reflecting prior beliefs regarding the parameters, for example, a meta-analysis of the effect of aspirin on the risk of a heart attack could provide the mean for a prior distribution of a regression parameter in a new study. For the most part, the choice of the prior is often made for mathematical convenience. Parameterized distributions are selected based on analytical considerations. For instance, a conjugate prior distribution combines nicely with the sampling distribution in that the posterior distribution only updates the parameters of the prior. Thus, when using conjugate priors, the data only modify the parameters of the prior distribution (and not the probability distribution). Variance components must be positive; therefore, parametric distributions restricted to positive values are only possible. Non-informative prior distributions are meant to reflect ignorance, such as placing the same probability for each possible value of the parameter using a uniform distribution.

While a meaningful discussion of the choices of a prior distribution is beyond the focus of this book, Table 24.1 provides a typology of possible prior distributions.

Table 24.1 Types of prior distributions.

Category	Feature
Subjective	Uses information from prior studies or elicited from experts. Can select a prior subject to moment constraints (e.g., maximum entropy)
Conjugate	Mathematically combines nicely with the sampling distribution, changing only the parameters but not the distribution.
Noninformative	Provides little information; depends on the scale of the parameter. Can be automatically generated (e.g., Jeffreys prior).
Improper	Simple to specify but does not integrate to one. Consequently, when combined with the likelihood, it may not lead to a proper posterior distribution.

2 The empirical Bayes analyst uses $m(y)$ to estimate θ. See Box 24.1.

The types of priors described are not mutually exclusive. For instance, subjective information may be used to construct a conjugate prior distribution.

The formula for the posterior distribution is explicit and always the same. However, in practice, it may not lead to a recognizable distribution, particularly in multi-parameter problems. Inferences are based on summaries of the posterior distribution, such as moments of the joint posterior distribution or marginal densities of parameters. The highest posterior regions and credible intervals for the parameters provide interval estimates, while hypothesis tests use Bayes factors.

24.2 Inference for HLM

24.2.1 Maximum Likelihood for the HLM

We rewrite the hierarchical linear model as a

$$Y_{ij} = \mathbf{x}_{ij}\boldsymbol{\beta} + \mathbf{z}_{ij}\boldsymbol{\theta}_i + \epsilon_{ij} \text{ where } \boldsymbol{\theta}_i \sim N_Q(\mathbf{0}, G_{\boldsymbol{\tau}}) \tag{24.2}$$

for $j = 1, 2, \ldots, n_i$; $i = 1, 2, \ldots, I$, and we assume that $\mathbf{z}_{ij} \in \mathbf{x}_{ij}$. This latter assumption ensures that the mean of $\boldsymbol{\theta}_i$ is zero, making the model in Eq. (24.2) a linear mixed model. Assume $\boldsymbol{\beta}$ is a $P \times 1$ vector of fixed parameters corresponding to a $1 \times P$ vector of patient covariates, $\mathbf{x}_{ij}$; $\boldsymbol{\theta}_i$ is a $Q \times 1$ vector of random parameters corresponding to the $1 \times Q$ vector of patient covariates, $\mathbf{z}_{ij}$; and $G_{\boldsymbol{\tau}}$ describes a $Q \times Q$ covariance matrix for the random effects. The Stage I errors are $\epsilon_{ij} \sim N(0, \sigma^2)$ and assume $\mathbb{E}(\epsilon_{ij}, \epsilon_{ij}^{\top}) = 0$ and the ϵ_{ij}s are independent of the components of $G_{\boldsymbol{\tau}}$. The linear mixed model can be written succinctly as

$$\underbrace{\mathbf{Y}_i}_{n_i\times 1} = \underbrace{X_i}_{n_i\times P}\boldsymbol{\beta} + \underbrace{Z_i}_{n_i\times Q}\boldsymbol{\theta}_i + \boldsymbol{\epsilon}_i \text{ where } \underbrace{\boldsymbol{\epsilon}_i}_{n_i\times 1} \sim N_{n_i}(\mathbf{0}, \underbrace{\Sigma_i}_{n_i\times n_i}) \text{ and } \underbrace{\boldsymbol{\theta}_i}_{Q\times 1} \sim N_Q(\mathbf{0}, \underbrace{G_{\boldsymbol{\tau}}}_{Q\times Q})$$

letting $\sigma^2 I_{n_i} = \Sigma_i$ without loss of generality.

Integration over the random effects yields the marginal likelihood for $\mathbf{Y}_i$ which is $N_{n_i}(X_i\boldsymbol{\beta}, H_i)$ where $H_i = Z_i G_{\boldsymbol{\tau}} Z_i^{\top} + \Sigma_i$. The marginal log-likelihood with $n = \sum_i n_i$ is

$$L(\boldsymbol{\beta}, \boldsymbol{\tau}, \sigma^2 \mid \mathbf{Y}) = -\frac{1}{2}\left\{n\log(2\pi) + \sum_i^I \log|H_i^{-1}| + \sum_i^I (\mathbf{Y}_i - X_i\boldsymbol{\beta})^{\top} H_i^{-1}(\mathbf{Y}_i - X_i\boldsymbol{\beta})\right\}.$$

To derive the maximum likelihood estimators, take partial derivatives of the log-likelihood for $\boldsymbol{\beta}$ and set it to 0 which yields

$$\hat{\boldsymbol{\beta}} = \left(\sum_{i=1}^I X_i^{\top}\widehat{H}_i^{-1}X_i\right)^{-1}\left(\sum_{i=1}^I X_i^{\top}\widehat{H}_i^{-1}\mathbf{Y}_i\right). \tag{24.3}$$

Because the estimator depends on the unknown parameters contained in H, estimates for $G_{\boldsymbol{\tau}}$ and σ^2 are substituted into the equation. The variance of $\widehat{\boldsymbol{\beta}}$ is

$$\text{Var}(\widehat{\boldsymbol{\beta}}) = \left(\sum_{i=1}^I X_i^{\top}\widehat{H}_i^{-1}X_i\right)^{-1}.$$

Statistical inference for $\boldsymbol{\beta}$ when comparing two nested models, such as a model with and without interaction terms, uses a likelihood ratio test based on the marginal log-likelihood. For instance, $L(m)$, for two different nested models, $m = 0, 1$, the test statistic is

$$-2(L(0) - L(1)) \sim \chi^2_k, \tag{24.4}$$

where k is the number of extra parameters in model 1 relative to model 0. In this test, the variance structure must be the same between the two models. Confidence intervals are constructed assuming the MLE is Normally distributed (see Eq. 24.1). An attractive feature of the likelihood ratio is its invariance to one-to-one transformations of the data. This means that the ratio is the same; that is, the likelihoods contain the same amount of information for the unknown parameters for different transformations of the data.

24.2.1.1 Estimation of Random Effects

The estimator of $\boldsymbol{\theta}_i$ can be motivated as minimizing the mean square error, $\mathbb{E}(\widehat{\boldsymbol{\theta}}_i - \boldsymbol{\theta}_i)^2$, and substituting $\widehat{\boldsymbol{\beta}}$ for $\boldsymbol{\beta}$,

$$\widehat{\boldsymbol{\theta}}_i = \mathbb{E}(\boldsymbol{\theta}_i \mid \mathbf{y}) \mid \boldsymbol{\beta} = \widehat{\boldsymbol{\beta}}) = \left(\sum_{i=1}^{I} Z_i^{\top} \Sigma_i^{-1} Z_i + G_{\boldsymbol{\tau}}^{-1}\right)^{-1} \sum_{i=1}^{I} Z_i^{\top} \Sigma_i^{-1} (\mathbf{Y}_i - X_i \widehat{\boldsymbol{\beta}}) \,. \tag{24.5}$$

Note that $\widehat{\theta}_i$ is not the maximum likelihood estimator of $\boldsymbol{\theta}_i$; it is the best linear unbiased estimator (BLUE) for $\mathbb{E}(\boldsymbol{\theta}_i \mid \mathbf{y})$ or the best linear unbiased predictor (BLUP) for $\boldsymbol{\theta}_i$.[3] The estimator is also the empirical Bayes estimator (see Box 24.1) for θ_i.

The variance of $\widehat{\boldsymbol{\theta}}_i$ is

$$\mathbf{v}_i = \mathrm{Var}(\widehat{\boldsymbol{\theta}}_i) = \left(\sum_{i=1}^{I} Z_i^{\top} \Sigma^{-1} Z_i + G_{\boldsymbol{\tau}}^{-1}\right)^{-1} \tag{24.6}$$

when interest centers on $\mathbb{E}(\boldsymbol{\theta}_i \mid \mathbf{y})$. Inference for the random effects proceeds using a Normal distribution. For instance, a $(1 - \alpha)$ confidence interval for θ_i is

$$\widehat{\theta}_i \pm z_{\frac{\alpha}{2}} \sqrt{v_{ii}}$$

Box 24.1 Empirical Bayes

Empirical Bayes uses the marginal likelihood $m(y \mid \boldsymbol{\tau})$ to estimate the parameters governing the distribution of the random effects, $\boldsymbol{\tau}$. This estimator is then used to construct an estimator for the remaining parameters, $p(\boldsymbol{\theta}, \boldsymbol{\beta}, \widehat{\boldsymbol{\tau}} \mid \mathbf{y}, X_i, Z_i)$. The estimator of $\boldsymbol{\tau}$ could be obtained using a method-of-moments approach or via marginal maximum likelihood. In the HLM, a key parameter of interest is the conditional parameter, $\mathbb{E}(\boldsymbol{\theta}_i \mid \mathbf{y})$ and its Empirical Bayes estimator is defined in Eq. (24.5). The uncertainty in the estimation of $\boldsymbol{\beta}$ and of the variance components $(\boldsymbol{\tau}, \sigma^2)$ are ignored although corrections for estimation of $\boldsymbol{\tau}$ have been suggested [75, 122]. We refer the reader to the book by Carlin and Louis [82] that provides a thorough treatment of empirical Bayes approaches.

[3] $\widehat{\theta}_i$ is described as a predictor because classical *likelihood* is defined for fixed parameters only.

with $z_{\frac{\alpha}{2}}$ selected is the upper $\alpha/2$ quantile from the standard Normal distribution, and v_{ii} is the ith diagonal component of $\mathbf{v}_i$. Because the plug-in estimates are used, and their uncertainty is ignored, the confidence interval is too narrow.

24.2.1.2 The REML

Restricted maximum likelihood (REML) is used to estimate the variance components of the HLM because the MLE of σ^2 is biased. REML maximizes the likelihood of a set of linearly independent error contrasts defined by the residuals $\mathbf{E}_i = \mathbf{Y}_i - X_i\widehat{\boldsymbol{\beta}}$. The REML maximizes $E_i{}^\top \mathbf{Y}_i$ rather than the likelihood for $\mathbf{Y}_i$ where $E_i^\top$ is an $(n_i - P) \times n_i$ matrix containing $n_i \times P$ linearly independent rows of $I_{n_i} - X_i(X_i^\top X_i)^{-1} X_i^\top$. Consequently, $E_i{}^\top \mathbf{Y}_i \sim N_{n_i}(\mathbf{0}, E_i^\top H_i E_i)$ in the HLM. The REML log-likelihood, ignoring the constant, is

$$L_R(\sigma^2, \boldsymbol{\tau} \mid E_i^\top \mathbf{Y}_i, \widehat{\boldsymbol{\beta}}) \propto -\frac{1}{2}\left\{\sum_{i=1}^{I} \log|H_i| + \sum_{i} \log|X_i^\top H_i^{-1} X_i| + \sum_{i=1}^{I} \mathbf{Y}_i^\top S_i \mathbf{Y}_i\right\}, \tag{24.7}$$

where $S_i = E_i(E_i^\top H_i^{-1} E_i)E_i^\top$ and $H_i = Z_i G_\tau Z_i^\top + \Sigma_i$. Differentiating with respect to σ^2 and the components of $\boldsymbol{\tau}$ yields

$$\widehat{\sigma}^2 = \frac{1}{n-P}\sum_{i=1}^{I} \mathbf{Y}_i^\top S_i \mathbf{Y}_i, \tag{24.8}$$

which again needs to be solved iteratively because the solution depends on the components of $G_{\boldsymbol{\tau}}$. Similarly, the REML estimator for $G_{\boldsymbol{\tau}}$ must be solved iteratively [123].

Inference for the variance parameters for models with different variance parameters but the same fixed effects using REML can be tested using a likelihood ratio test,

$$-2(L_R(0) - L_R(1)) \sim \chi_k^2. \tag{24.9}$$

While the test statistic is asymptotically χ_k^2, because the null hypothesis that $G_\tau^2 = 0$ is on the boundary of the parameter space, standard asymptotic theory no longer holds. A mixture of χ^2 distributions has been proposed when testing this hypothesis.[4]

24.2.2 Extended Maximum Likelihood for the HLM

The likelihood principle was expanded [124] to show that an *extended likelihood* function includes all the information in the data for both fixed and random parameters. Lee and Nelder [79] demonstrated how to use the extended likelihood in the setting of hierarchical generalized linear models.

[4] It is worth noting that it is unlikely that $\tau^2 = 0$—the question is whether the variance is small enough to safely ignore.

The extended log-likelihood of the joint parameters can be partitioned into two pieces,

$$L_e(\boldsymbol{\beta}, \boldsymbol{\theta}_i, \sigma^2, \boldsymbol{\tau} \mid \mathbf{Y}_i) = \underbrace{L_{e_1}(\boldsymbol{\beta}, \sigma^2, \boldsymbol{\tau} \mid \mathbf{Y}_i)}_{\text{marginal likelihood}} + \underbrace{L_{e_2}(\boldsymbol{\theta}_i \mid \boldsymbol{\tau}, \sigma^2, \boldsymbol{\beta}, \mathbf{Y}_i)}_{\text{conditional likelihood}}, \tag{24.10}$$

where the subscript e denotes extended likelihood. In the extended likelihood, $\exp(L_{e_2})$ is referred to as the predictive probability for the random effects. If the scale of the random effects (or a linear function of the random effects) is additive to the fixed effects (denoted *canonical or weak canonical* scale), then the extended likelihood is denoted a *hierarchical likelihood* (h-likelihood). If the extended likelihood is **not** an h-likelihood, then estimation proceeds as follows:

1. Use the marginal likelihood to obtain an estimate of $\boldsymbol{\beta}$.
2. Use the extended likelihood, given the values of $\boldsymbol{\beta}$, to derive the MLE for $\boldsymbol{\theta}_i$.
3. Use REML, given the values of $\boldsymbol{\beta}$ and $\boldsymbol{\theta}_i$, to derive estimates for σ^2 and $G_{\boldsymbol{\tau}}$.

If the extended likelihood is an h-likelihood, joint maximization of the h-likelihood provides estimators for all parameters. Moreover,

1. The estimator of $\boldsymbol{\beta}$ that maximizes the marginal likelihood is the same as the estimator that maximizes the h-likelihood.
2. The Fisher Information matrix for the marginal likelihood is the same as the relevant component from the h-likelihood.
3. The variance of $\boldsymbol{\theta}_i$ obtained from the Fisher Information matrix via the h-likelihood accounts for the uncertainty in the estimation of $\boldsymbol{\beta}$.

Box 24.2 Estimating fixed effects and variance components for the HLM

1. Start with initial estimates $G_{(0)}$ and $\Sigma_{(0)}$.[a]
2. Solve for $\boldsymbol{\beta}^{(0)}$ and $\boldsymbol{\theta}_i^{(0)}$,

$$\left(\sum_{i=1}^{I} X_i^{\top}\Sigma_{(0)}^{-1}X_i\right)\boldsymbol{\beta}^{(0)} = \sum_{i=1}^{I} X_i^{\top}\Sigma_{(0)}^{-1}X_i(\mathbf{Y}_i - Z^{\top}\boldsymbol{\theta}_i^{(0)}), \tag{24.11}$$

$$\left(\sum_{i=1}^{I} Z_i^{\top}\Sigma_{(0)}^{-1}X_iZ_i + G_{(0)}^{-1}\right)\boldsymbol{\theta}_i^{(0)} = \sum_{i=1}^{I} Z_i^{\top}\Sigma_{(0)}^{-1}X_i(\mathbf{Y}_i - X_i^{\top}\boldsymbol{\beta}_i^{(0)}). \tag{24.12}$$

3. Using $\widehat{\boldsymbol{\beta}}^{(0)}$, maximize the REML log-likelihood

$$-\frac{1}{2}\left\{\sum_{i=1}^{I}\log|H_i| + \sum_{i}\log|X_i^{\top}H_i^{-1}X_i| + \sum_{i=1}^{I}\mathbf{Y}_i^{\top}S_i\mathbf{Y}_i\right\}, \tag{24.13}$$

where $H_i = Z_iG_{\boldsymbol{\tau}}Z_i^{\top} + \Sigma$ and $S_i = E_i(E_i^{\top}H_i^{-1}E_i)E_i^{\top}$, to obtain $G_{(1)}$ and $\Sigma_{(1)}$.
4. Repeat until convergence.

[a] We have dropped the "i" subscript on Σ_i.

Returning to the HLM, the random effects ($\boldsymbol{\theta}_i$) are additive to the linear predictor so that the extended likelihood is an h-log-likelihood,

$$L_h = -\frac{1}{2}\left\{\log \mid 2\pi\Sigma_i \mid + \frac{1}{2}\sum_{i=1}^{I}(\mathbf{Y}_i - X_i\boldsymbol{\beta} - Z_i\boldsymbol{\theta}_i)^\top \Sigma_i^{-1}(\mathbf{Y}_i - X_i\boldsymbol{\beta} - Z_i\boldsymbol{\theta}_i)\right.$$
$$\left. + \log \mid 2\pi G_{\boldsymbol{\tau}} \mid + \sum_{i=1}^{I}\boldsymbol{\theta}_i^\top G_{\boldsymbol{\tau}}^{-1}\boldsymbol{\theta}_i\right\}, \qquad (24.14)$$

so that joint maximization of the h-likelihood can be used. The estimators solve

$$\begin{pmatrix} \sum_{i=1}^{I} X_i^\top \Sigma_i^{-1} X_i & \sum_{i=1}^{I} X_i^\top \Sigma_i^{-1} Z_i \\ \sum_{i=1}^{I} Z_i^\top \Sigma_i^{-1} X_i & \sum_{i=1}^{I} Z_i^\top \Sigma_i^{-1} Z_i + G_{\boldsymbol{\tau}}^{-1} \end{pmatrix} \begin{pmatrix} \widehat{\boldsymbol{\beta}} \\ \widehat{\boldsymbol{\theta}}_i \end{pmatrix} = \begin{pmatrix} \sum_{i=1}^{I} X_i^\top \Sigma_i^{-1} \mathbf{Y}_i \\ \sum_{i=1}^{I} Z_i^\top \Sigma_i^{-1} \mathbf{Y}_i \end{pmatrix} \qquad (24.15)$$

and yield the MLE for $\boldsymbol{\beta}$ and the BLUP for $\boldsymbol{\theta}_i$. The estimators for Σ_i and $G_{\boldsymbol{\tau}}$ use REML. Confidence intervals and tests utilize likelihood ratios as described in the marginal maximum likelihood and REML methods discussed earlier. Letting

$$A = \begin{pmatrix} \sum_{i=1}^{I} X_i^\top \Sigma_i^{-1} X_i & \sum_{i=1}^{I} X_i^\top \Sigma_i^{-1} Z_i \\ \sum_{i=1}^{I} Z_i^\top \Sigma_i^{-1} X_i & \sum_{i=1}^{I} Z_i^\top \Sigma_i^{-1} Z_i + G_{\boldsymbol{\tau}}^{-1} \end{pmatrix}$$

then the (unconditional) variance of $\boldsymbol{\theta}_i$ taken from A^{-1} accounts for the uncertainty in using $\boldsymbol{\beta}$ and is given by

$$\mathrm{Var}(\widehat{\boldsymbol{\theta}}_i) = \sum_i \Omega_i^{-1} Z_i^\top \Sigma_i^{-1} X_i \left(\sum_i X_i^\top H_i X_i\right)^{-1} X_i^\top \Sigma_i^{-1} Z_i \Omega_i^{-1}, \qquad (24.16)$$

where $\Omega_i = Z_i^\top \Sigma_i^{-1} Z_i + G_{\boldsymbol{\tau}}^{-1}$. Compare Eq. (24.6) that ignores the uncertainty in $\boldsymbol{\beta}$ and 24.16 which does not. Box 24.2 summarizes the approach to estimation using the h-likelihood for the HLM.

24.2.3 Iterative Weighted Least Squares

Iterative weighted least squares (IWLS) can be used for obtaining estimates. Box 24.3 describes the algorithm that becomes particularly useful for the HGLM.

In the HLM, $\phi = \sigma^2$, $V(\mu_{ij}) = 1$, $\rho = \tau^2$, $V_\theta(\boldsymbol{\theta}_i) = 1$, with

$$\boldsymbol{\delta} = \begin{pmatrix} \boldsymbol{\beta}^\top \\ \boldsymbol{\theta}_i^\top \end{pmatrix}; \text{ and } \Sigma_a = \begin{pmatrix} \Sigma_i & 0 \\ 0 & G_{\boldsymbol{\tau}} \end{pmatrix}.$$

24.2.4 Bayesian Approaches for the HLM

The Bayesian does not distinguish between fixed and random effects, as all parameters are assumed to be random. Re-express Eq. (24.2) as

$$\begin{aligned} Y_{ij} \mid \boldsymbol{\alpha}_i, \sigma^2 &= \mathbf{x}_{ij}\boldsymbol{\alpha}_i + \epsilon_{ij};\ \epsilon_{ij} \sim N(0, \sigma^2), \\ \boldsymbol{\alpha}_i \mid \boldsymbol{\mu}, G_{\boldsymbol{\tau}} &= \boldsymbol{\mu} + \boldsymbol{\omega}_i;\ \boldsymbol{\omega}_i \sim N_Q(\mathbf{0}, G_{\boldsymbol{\tau}}) \end{aligned}$$

and prior distributions for σ^2, $\boldsymbol{\mu}$, and $G_{\boldsymbol{\tau}}^{-1}$ are required. Assume

Box 24.3 Iterative weighted least squares

Let $\mathbb{E}(y) = \mu$, $\text{var}(y) = \phi V(\mu)$, $\mathbb{E}(\psi_r) = r$, and $\text{var}(\psi_r) = \rho V_r(r)$. Define $\eta_a = (\eta^\top, \eta_r^\top) = T\boldsymbol{\delta}$ where $\eta = l(\mu) = \mathbf{X}\boldsymbol{\beta} + \mathbf{Z}v$ and $\eta_r = l_r(r) = v$. Stack the fixed and random effects such that

$$\boldsymbol{\delta} = \begin{pmatrix} \boldsymbol{\beta}^\top \\ v^\top \end{pmatrix}; \text{ and } T = \begin{pmatrix} X & Z \\ 0 & I \end{pmatrix}.$$

Given (ϕ, ρ), $\boldsymbol{\delta}$ can be estimated by solving the iterative weighted least squares equation

$$(T^\top \Sigma_a^{-1} T)^{-1}\widehat{\boldsymbol{\delta}} = T^\top \Sigma_a^{-1} \boldsymbol{\omega}_a \text{ with} \qquad (24.17)$$

$$\boldsymbol{\omega}_a = \begin{pmatrix} \boldsymbol{\omega}_L^\top \\ \boldsymbol{\omega}_{ri}^\top \end{pmatrix}; \ \Sigma_a = \Gamma W_a^{-1}; \ \Gamma = \text{diag}(\boldsymbol{\phi}, \boldsymbol{\rho}); \ \boldsymbol{\phi} = \text{diag}(\phi_i); \ \boldsymbol{\rho} = \text{diag}(\rho_i).$$

The matrix $W_a = \text{diag}(W_y, W_r)$ contains weights that will be iteratively updated. Let μ^0, r_i^0, ϕ^0, and ρ^0 denote starting values, and note that ψ_r takes the value determined by the constraint on $\mathbb{E}(r_i)$. The algorithm proceeds as follows:

1. Create the adjusted dependent variables and weight matrices
   (a) Compute $\boldsymbol{\omega}_i = \eta_i^0 + (\mathbf{Y}_i - \mu_i^0)\left(\frac{\partial \eta_i}{\partial \mu_i}\right)_{\mu=\mu^0}$ and $\boldsymbol{\omega}_{ri} = v_i^0 + (\psi_r - r_i^0)\left(\frac{\partial v_i}{\partial r_i}\right)_{r_i=r_i^0}$.
   (b) Compute $W_y = \left(\frac{\partial \mu_i}{\partial \eta_i}\right)^2_{\mu_i=\mu_i^0} V(\mu_i^0)^{-1}$ and $W_r = \left(\frac{\partial r_i}{\partial v_i}\right)^2_{r_i=r_i^0} V(r_i^0)^{-1}$.
2. Solve for $\boldsymbol{\delta}$ in Eq. (24.17) to get updated estimates, μ_i^1 and r_i^1.
3. Using μ_i^1 and r_i^1, re-estimate ϕ and ρ using REML.
4. Repeat 1–3 until differences in values between iteration k and $k+1$ are small.

Table 24.2 Prior distributions for parameters in the HLM.

Distribution of X	Parameters	Mean; variance
Normal	$-\infty < X, \mu < \infty$	$\mathbb{E}(X) = \mu$
$X \sim N(\mu, \sigma^2)$	scale $\sigma > 0$	$\text{Var}(X) = \sigma^2$
Inverse Gamma	$X > 0$; scale $\beta > 0$	$\mathbb{E}(X) = \frac{\beta}{\alpha-1}$, $\alpha > 1$
$X \sim \text{Inv-Gamma}(\alpha, \beta)$	shape $\alpha > 0$	$\text{Var}(X) = \frac{\beta^2}{(\alpha-1)^2(\alpha-2)}$; $\alpha > 2$
Wishart	X, R : symmetric positive definite	$\mathbb{E}(X_{ij}) = \nu R_{ij}$
$X_{k\times k} \sim \text{Wishart}(R_{k\times k}, \nu)$	$\nu > 0$	$\text{Var}(X_{ij}) = \nu(R_{ij}^2 + R_{ii}R_{jj})$

$$\boldsymbol{\mu} \sim N_Q(\mathbf{c}, D), \ \sigma^2 \sim \text{Inv-Gamma}(a, b), \text{ and } G_{\boldsymbol{\tau}}^{-1} \sim \text{Wishart}([dR]^{-1}, d). \qquad (24.18)$$

Values for d, a, b, c, D, R^{-1}, and f must be specified. Features of these prior distributions are listed in Table 24.2. The mean of the provider-specific parameters, $\boldsymbol{\mu}$, is assumed to follow a multivariate normal distribution (dimension $= Q$) with expectation $\mathbf{c}$ and $Q \times Q$ symmetric positive definite variance matrix D. Because the conjugate prior distribution for σ^2 is the Inv-Gamma, we select it for the prior distribution. For a similar reason, the between-provider variance, $G_{\boldsymbol{\tau}}^{-1}$, is assumed to follow a Wishart distribution having degrees of freedom d and $Q \times Q$ symmetric positive definite scale matrix $(dR)^{-1}$. Note that Eq. (24.18) can include covariates that do not vary by cluster, for example, $Y_{ij} = \mathbf{x}_{ij}\boldsymbol{\beta} + \mathbf{z}_{ij}\boldsymbol{\theta}_i + \epsilon_{ij}$, and if so, prior distributions for the components of $\boldsymbol{\beta}$ are also required.

The joint posterior distribution for the parameters, $f(\boldsymbol{\alpha}_1, \ldots, \boldsymbol{\alpha}_I, \sigma^2, \boldsymbol{\mu}, G_{\boldsymbol{\tau}}^{-1} \mid \mathbf{Y})$, is

$$\propto f(\sigma^2 \mid a, b) f(\boldsymbol{\mu} \mid \mathbf{c}, D) f(G_{\boldsymbol{\tau}}^{-1} \mid R^{-1}, \nu) \prod_{i=1}^{I} \prod_{j=1}^{n_i} f(Y_{ij} \mid \boldsymbol{\alpha}_i, \sigma^2) f(\boldsymbol{\alpha}_i \mid \boldsymbol{\mu}, G_{\boldsymbol{\tau}}^{-1}).$$

The computational strategies described in Volume 2, Chapter 23, are used to compute the joint posterior distribution and summaries, such as the mean, median, and quantiles, of the posterior are used for inference. Suppose Gibbs sampling is used to estimate the posterior distribution. The full conditional distributions are required. Let $\mathbf{Y}_i = (Y_{i1}, Y_{i2}, \ldots, Y_{in_i})^\top$ and $\mathbf{x}_i = n_i \times Q$ design matrix with the first column a vector of ones. Denote all the parameters by Γ and all parameters except parameter $*$ by Γ_{-*}. We have

$$\boldsymbol{\alpha}_i \mid \Gamma_{-\boldsymbol{\alpha}_i}, \mathbf{Y} \sim N_Q(A_{\alpha_i} a_{\alpha_i}, A_{\alpha_i}), \text{ where } A_{\alpha_i} = \left(\frac{\mathbf{x}_i^\top \mathbf{x}_i}{\sigma^2} + G_{\boldsymbol{\tau}}^{-1} \right)^{-1},$$

$$a_{\alpha_i} = \left(\frac{\mathbf{x}_i^\top \mathbf{Y}_i}{\sigma^2} + G_{\boldsymbol{\tau}}^{-1} \boldsymbol{\alpha}_i \right) \text{ for } i = 1, 2, \ldots, I.$$

Write the Stage II model as

$$\underbrace{\begin{pmatrix} \boldsymbol{\alpha}_1 \\ \boldsymbol{\alpha}_2 \\ \vdots \\ \boldsymbol{\alpha}_I \end{pmatrix}}_{\tilde{\boldsymbol{\alpha}}} = \underbrace{\begin{pmatrix} I_Q \\ I_Q \\ \vdots \\ I_Q \end{pmatrix}}_{\tilde{I}} \boldsymbol{\mu} + \underbrace{\begin{pmatrix} \boldsymbol{\omega}_1 \\ \boldsymbol{\omega}_2 \\ \vdots \\ \boldsymbol{\omega}_I \end{pmatrix}}_{\tilde{\boldsymbol{\omega}}}$$

where I_Q is the $Q \times Q$ identity matrix, and recall that $\boldsymbol{\mu} \sim N_Q(\mathbf{c}, D)$ so that

$$\boldsymbol{\mu} \mid \Gamma_{-\boldsymbol{\mu}}, \mathbf{Y} \sim N_Q(A_{\boldsymbol{\mu}} a_{\boldsymbol{\mu}}, A_{\boldsymbol{\mu}}) \text{ with } A_{\boldsymbol{\mu}} = (I \times G_{\boldsymbol{\tau}}^{-1} + D^{-1})^{-1},$$

$$a_{\boldsymbol{\mu}} = \left(I \times G_{\boldsymbol{\tau}}^{-1} \bar{\boldsymbol{\alpha}} + D^{-1} \mathbf{c} \right) \text{ where } \bar{\boldsymbol{\alpha}} = \frac{1}{I} \sum_{i=1}^{I} \boldsymbol{\alpha}_i.$$

With $\sigma^2 \sim \text{Inv-Gamma}(a, b)$, the full conditional distribution for σ^2 is

$$\sigma^2 \mid \Gamma_{-\sigma^2}, \mathbf{Y} \sim \text{Inverse-Gamma} \left(\frac{\sum_i n_i}{2} + a, \left[\frac{1}{2} \sum_{i=1}^{I} (\mathbf{Y}_i - \mathbf{x}_i \boldsymbol{\alpha}_i)^\top (\mathbf{Y}_i - \mathbf{x}_i \boldsymbol{\alpha}_i) + b^{-1} \right]^{-1} \right).$$

Last, the full conditional for $G_{\boldsymbol{\tau}}^{-1}$ assuming $G_{\boldsymbol{\tau}}^{-1} \sim \text{Wishart}([\nu R]^{-1}, \nu)$ is

$$G_{\boldsymbol{\tau}}^{-1} \mid \Gamma_{-G_{\boldsymbol{\tau}}}, \mathbf{Y} \sim \text{Wishart} \left(\left[\sum_{i=1}^{I} (\boldsymbol{\alpha}_i - \boldsymbol{\mu})(\boldsymbol{\alpha}_i - \boldsymbol{\mu})^\top + \nu R \right]^{-1}, \sum_{i=1}^{I} n_i + \nu \right).$$

Table 24.3 Draws of $\Gamma = (\alpha_i, \mu, \sigma^2, G_\tau)$ using the Gibbs sampler.

	Iterations						
Chain	1	2	$\cdots$	t	$t+1$	$\cdots$	$t+m$
1	$\Gamma_1^{(0)}$	$\Gamma_1^{(1)}$	$\cdots$	$\Gamma_1^{(t)}$	$\Gamma_1^{(t+1)}$	$\cdots$	$\Gamma_1^{(t+m)}$
2	$\Gamma_2^{(0)}$	$\Gamma_2^{(1)}$	$\cdots$	$\Gamma_2^{(t)}$	$\Gamma_2^{(t+1)}$	$\cdots$	$\Gamma_2^{(t+m)}$
$\vdots$	$\vdots$	$\vdots$	$\vdots$	$\vdots$	$\vdots$	$\vdots$	$\vdots$
S	$\Gamma_S^{(0)}$	$\Gamma_S^{(1)}$	$\cdots$	$\Gamma_S^{tm)}$	$\Gamma_S^{(t+1)}$	$\cdots$	$\Gamma_S^{(t+m)}$
	Burn-in				For Inference		

The full conditional distributions all arise from known densities from which it is easy to sample.

Inference is based on summaries of draws $t+1$ to $t+m$ from chains 1 to S of Γ, assuming the sampler has converged by iteration t (Table 24.3). For instance,

$$\widehat{\alpha}_i = \frac{1}{S}\sum_{k=1}^{S}\frac{1}{m}\sum_{l=1}^{m}\alpha_k^{(t+l)}.$$

24.3 Hospital Satisfaction HLM Example

We revisit the hospital satisfaction data introduced in Volume 2, Chapter 20, "Introduction to Hierarchical Linear Models," where Y_{ij} is a patient-reported satisfaction score measured at hospital discharge and $\mathbf{x}_{ij}$ includes patient age at hospital admission, sex, and a measure of admission severity. There are 1,977 patients treated at 20 hospitals. Higher values of Y_{ij} correspond to higher satisfaction, and higher values of the severity score correspond to sicker patients. The GLLM version of the model is

$$Y_{ij} = \beta_0 + \beta_1\text{Age}_{ij} + \beta_2\text{Female}_{ij} + \beta_3\text{Severity}_{ij} + r_i + \epsilon_{ij},\ r_i \sim N(0, \tau^2)$$

and $\epsilon_{ij} \sim N(0, \sigma^2)$. Three different approaches are used to estimate the parameters (see Box 24.4). The first uses the R function lmer that is based on classical likelihood for estimation of the regression coefficients, BLUPs for the hospital random effects, and REML for the variance components. Adaptive Gaussian quadrature is used for integration. For extended likelihood, the R package hglm is used for the random effects using the h-likelihood, the marginal likelihood for the regression coefficients, and REML for the variance components. Computation in hglm uses extended quasi-likelihood (EQL) implemented via iterative weighted least squares.[5]

[5] EQL for HGLMs uses estimating equations for two interlinked GLMs: one for the mean (including fixed and random effects) and one for the variance components.

Box 24.4 R code for patient satisfaction via HLM

```
Classical Likelihood
lmer(outcomes ~  (1|hosp.id) + cage + female + cseverity,
     data=lindata.set)
Extended Likelihood
hglm((fixed=outcomes ~ cage + female + cseverity,random = ~ 1|hosp.id,
   data=lindata.set)
Bayesian
apar <- 0.001; bpar <- 0.01
lgprior <- list(prec = list(prior="loggamma", param = c(apar,bpar)))
formula = outcomes ~ cage+ female + cseverity + f(hosp.id, model="iid",
   hyper = lgprior)
result <- inla(formula, family="gaussian",data=lindata.set)
```

We assume mutually independent priors for $\beta_p, p = 0, 1, 2, 3$, arising from $N(0, 1{,}000)$ (INLA default), and both σ^2 and τ^2 arise from log-gamma distribution using Gamma(0.001, 0.01). The INLA default prior distribution for variance components uses Gamma(1, 0.00001).

Table 24.4 HLM estimates (standard errors) obtained using classical likelihood, extended likelihood, and fully Bayesian approaches. Bayesian values are posterior means and posterior standard deviations.

Parameter	Simulated values	Likelihood-based classical	Likelihood-based extended	Posterior mean (SD)
Intercept	50	51.49 (0.750)	51.48 (0.762)	51.49 (0.783)
Age, centered	0.50	0.55 (0.045)	0.55 (0.045)	0.55 (0.045)
Female	−1.20	−1.61(0.965)	−1.61(0.965)	−1.61(0.965)
Severity, centered	2.50	2.60 (0.445)	2.60 (0.445)	2.60 (0.445)
σ^2	400	381.62	381.56	381.56
τ^2	4	4.61	4.77	4.56

Fully Bayesian estimates are obtained using the INLA package called from R. Computation in INLA is based on a set of nested Laplace approximations [125].

Table 24.4 presents the estimates using the three different approaches. The point estimates are in close agreement; the standard errors from the extended likelihood standard errors and the posterior standard deviations are equal to or larger than those from the classical likelihood. The Bayesian approach provides estimated marginal densities for various parameters of interest. Figure 24.1 displays the estimated posterior distributions for σ^2 and τ^2 obtained from the function INLA as well as the estimated density for the intra-class correlation coefficient (ICC). The density for τ^2 has a long right tail; the median value is 3.66, and the upper quartile is 6.36. The posterior mean ICC is 1.2%, suggesting a small hospital signal. Also displayed are the estimates of 5 randomly selected hospital random effects, $\widehat{r}_i$. Values of $\widehat{r}_i < 0$ correspond to a decrease in hospital satisfaction. For instance, hospital A is shifted left of 0.

Figure 24.1 Marginal posterior densities for variance components, ICC, and hospital random effects: patient satisfaction data.

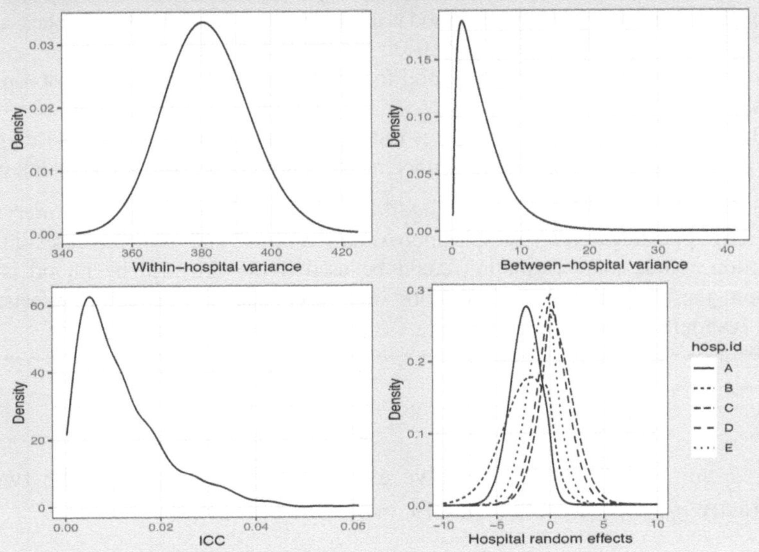

24.4 Inference for the HGLM

24.4.1 Extended Maximum Likelihood for the HGLM

Recall from Volume 2, Chapter 21, that the HGLM can be represented as a Generalized Linear Mixed Model (GLMM). Let $\eta_{ij} = l(\mathbb{E}(Y_{ij} \mid \boldsymbol{\theta}_i))$.

1. Conditional on the random effects, r_i, the outcomes arise from a GLM in which the log-likelihood is proportional to

$$\sum_{i=1}^{I}\sum_{j=1}^{n_i}\left\{\frac{y_{ij}\theta_{ij} - b(\theta_{ij}) + c(y_{ij})}{\phi}\right\} \quad \text{where } \eta_{ij} = l(\mu_{ij}) = \sum_k \beta_k x_{kij} + z_{kij}v_i.$$

   $\mathbb{E}(y_{ij} \mid r_i) = \mu_{ij}$, $\text{Var}(y_{ij} \mid r_i) = \phi V(\mu_{ij})$, and $v_i = v(r_i)$ is a monotone function of r_i.
2. The random effects follow a distribution conjugate to the GLM. Thus, r_i has log-density from a one-parameter exponential distribution proportional to

$$\sum_{i=1}^{I}\frac{\psi_R\theta_R(r_i) - b_R(\theta_R(r_i))}{\lambda}, \tag{24.19}$$

   where $\mathbb{E}(r_i) = \psi_R$, $\text{Var}(r_i) = \rho\text{V}(\psi_R)$, and λ is a dispersion parameter.
3. Constraint: select the value of $\mathbb{E}(r_i)$ such that $v(r_i) = 0$.

Box 24.5 describes the algorithm for obtaining parameter estimates. Likelihood ratio tests can be used to compare nested models, whereas the Akaike information criterion is used for non-nested models. These issues are further discussed in the next chapter. As in the HLM, iterative weighted least squares for an augmented

Box 24.5 Inference using h-Likelihood

1. Use the h-likelihood for inferences for v_i.
2. Use the marginal likelihood for inferences for β_k.
   (a) When the marginal log-likelihood is numerically intractable, use a Laplace approximation replacing the random effects by their estimates.
3. Use the restricted maximum likelihood to get inferences about the dispersion parameters, ϕ, and λ.
   (a) When the restricted likelihood is numerically intractable, use a Laplace approximation replacing the fixed parameters and random effects with their estimates.

Point estimates are obtained by solving the score equations; confidence intervals are obtained by appealing to large-sample approximation theory and using the observed Fisher information. While joint estimation could be used if the extended likelihood is an h-likelihood, the algorithm above will work when the scale of the random effects is not (weakly) canonical.

linear predictor can be used to derive estimators for $\boldsymbol{\beta}$ and r_i. The two linear predictors are $\eta_{ij} = X_{ij}\boldsymbol{\beta} + Z_i\boldsymbol{\theta}_i$ and $\eta_{R_i} = \boldsymbol{v}_i$. See Box 24.3.

24.4.2 Bayesian Approaches for the HGLM

Suppose we adopt the GLLM formulation so that conditional on the cluster effects, $\boldsymbol{\theta}_i$,

$$p(y_{ij} \mid r_i) \propto \exp\left(\frac{y_{ij}\theta_{ij} - b(\theta_{ij}) + c(y_{ij})}{\phi}\right) \tag{24.20}$$

with $\mathbb{E}(y_{ij} \mid r_i) = \mu_{ij}$, $\eta_{ij} = l(\mu_{ij}) = \sum_k \beta_k x_{kij} + z_{kij} r_i$, and $\text{Var}(y_{ij} \mid r_i) = \phi V(\mu_{ij})$. Assuming the r_i's are independent with $\mathbb{E}(r_i) = 0$ and arise from a 1-parameter exponential family with variance $\rho V(\psi_R)$ and letting $\omega = (0, \rho V(\psi_R)$, then the posterior distribution is

$$f(r_1, \ldots, r_I, \boldsymbol{\beta}, \omega) \propto \left\{\prod_{i=1}^{I}\prod_{j=1}^{n_i} p(y_{ij} \mid \mathbf{x}_{ij}\boldsymbol{\beta})P(\boldsymbol{\beta})\right\}\left\{\prod_{i=1}^{I} P(r_i \mid \omega)P(\omega))\right\}. \tag{24.21}$$

The full conditionals (see Volume 2, Chapter 23, "Computational Approaches") are

$$\begin{aligned}
P\boldsymbol{\beta} \mid \mathbf{y}, \mathbf{r}, \omega) &\propto \prod_{i=1}^{I}\prod_{j=1}^{n_i} p(y_{ij} \mid \mathbf{x}_{ij}, r_i, \boldsymbol{\beta})P(\boldsymbol{\beta}),\\
P(r_i \mid \mathbf{y}, \mathbf{r}_{-\mathbf{i}}, \boldsymbol{\beta}, \omega) &\propto \prod_{i=1}^{I} P(y_{ij} \mid \boldsymbol{\beta}, r_i, x_{ij})P(r_i \mid \boldsymbol{\beta}),\\
\text{and } P(\omega \mid \mathbf{y}, \mathbf{r}, \boldsymbol{\beta}) &\propto \prod_{i=1}^{I} P(r_i \mid \omega)P(\omega).
\end{aligned}$$

24.5 Poisson Stage I and Gamma Stage II

Suppose we have I provides, each treating n_i subjects, with y_{ij} arising from a Poisson distribution

$$\mu_{ij} = \mathbb{E}(y_{ij} \mid r_i) = r_i \exp(\mathbf{x}_{ij}\boldsymbol{\beta}) \text{ and } \log \mu_{ij} = \mathbf{x}_{ij}\boldsymbol{\beta} + v_i \text{ with } v_i = \log r_i,$$

so that the random effect is additive on the log scale. Assume that r_i arises from a Gamma(λ) distribution where

$$f(r_i) = \frac{1}{\lambda}^{\frac{1}{\lambda}} r_i^{\frac{1}{\lambda}-1} \exp(-r_i/\lambda) \left(\frac{1}{\Gamma(1/\lambda)}\right), \ \lambda > 0,$$

where $\mathbb{E}(r_i)$ is set to 1. Because the random effect is additive on the log scale to the linear predictor, the extended likelihood is an h-likelihood, which we can jointly maximize to obtain parameter estimates of both the fixed and random effects.

24.5.1 Extended Likelihood

The Stage I contribution to the likelihood is

$$\log f(\mathbf{y}_i) \propto \sum_{j=1}^{n_i} \Big(y_{ij}(\mathbf{x}_{ij}\boldsymbol{\beta} + v_i - r_i \exp(\mathbf{x}_{ij}\boldsymbol{\beta})\Big).$$

To obtain the h-likelihood, we need $f(v_i)$, which requires multiplying $f(r_i)$ by the Jacobian of transformation from r_i to v_i, $J(r_i \to v_i) = r_i$. Thus, the Stage II contribution to the likelihood from cluster i is

$$\log f(v_i) \propto \left(\frac{v_i - r_i}{\lambda} - \frac{\log \lambda}{\lambda} - \log \Gamma\left(\frac{1}{\lambda}\right)\right).$$

The kernel of the h-likelihood is

$$\log h = \sum_{i=1}^{I} \sum_{j=1}^{n_i} \Big(y_{ij} \log \mu_{ij} - \mu_{ij}\Big) + \sum_{i=1}^{I} \left(\frac{v_i - r_i}{\lambda} - \frac{\log \lambda}{\lambda} - \log \Gamma\left(\frac{1}{\lambda}\right)\right).$$

Letting $y_{i+} = \sum_j y_{ij}$ and $\mu_{i+} = \sum_j \mu_{ij}$ yields

$$\frac{\partial \log h}{\partial v_i} = \left(y_{i+} + \frac{1}{\lambda}\right) - \left(\mu_{i+} + \frac{1}{\lambda}\right) r_i, \tag{24.22}$$

$$\frac{\partial \log h}{\partial \beta_k} = \sum_{i=1}^{I} \sum_{j=1}^{n_i} (y_{ij} - \mu_{ij}) x_{kij}. \tag{24.23}$$

Setting these to 0 and solving provides the MLE for β_k and the BLUP for r_i, for example,

$$\mathbb{E}(r_i \mid \mathbf{y}, \widehat{\mu}, \widehat{\lambda}) = \frac{y_{i+} + 1/\widehat{\lambda}}{\widehat{\mu}_{i+} + 1/\widehat{\lambda}}.$$

Note that Eq. (24.23) may be also expressed as

$$\frac{\partial \log h}{\partial \beta_k} = \sum_{i=1}^{I}\sum_{j=1}^{n_i}\left\{y_{ij} - \frac{\mu_{ij}}{\mu_{i+}}y_{i+} + \frac{\lambda\mu_{ij}}{\mu_{i+}(\mu_{i+}+\lambda)}(y_{i+} - \mu_{i+})\right\}x_{kij}, \quad (24.24)$$

which shows how the score equation for each β_k is a function of the within- and between-cluster information. Likelihood ratio tests are used to compare models.

24.5.2 Bayesian Inference

Referring to Eq. (24.21), the posterior distribution is

$$c\left\{\prod_{i=1}^{I}\prod_{j=1}^{n_i}\frac{(\mathbf{x}_{ij}\boldsymbol{\beta} + r_i)^{y_{ij}}}{y_{ij}!}e^{-(\mathbf{x}_{ij}\boldsymbol{\beta}+r_i)}P(\boldsymbol{\beta})\right\}\left\{\prod_{i=1}^{I}\frac{1}{\lambda}^{\frac{1}{\lambda}}r_i^{\frac{1}{\lambda}-1}e^{-\frac{r_i}{\lambda}}\left(\frac{1}{\Gamma(1/\lambda)}\right)P(\lambda))\right\}.$$

Prior distributions are required for the regression coefficients, $\boldsymbol{\beta}$, and for λ. Inference proceeds using Gibbs sampling based on the full conditional distributions:

$$\begin{aligned}
P\boldsymbol{\beta} \mid \mathbf{y}, \mathbf{r}, \lambda) &\propto P(\boldsymbol{\beta})\prod_{i=1}^{I}\prod_{j=1}^{n_i}p(y_{ij} \mid \mathbf{x}_{ij}, r_i, \boldsymbol{\beta}),\\
P(r_i \mid \mathbf{y}, r_{-i}, \boldsymbol{\beta}, \lambda) &\propto \prod_{i=1}^{I}P(y_{ij} \mid \boldsymbol{\beta}, r_i, x_{ij})P(r_i \mid \boldsymbol{\beta}),\\
\text{and } P(\lambda \mid \mathbf{y}, \mathbf{r}, \boldsymbol{\beta}) &\propto P(\lambda)\prod_{i=1}^{I}\frac{1}{\lambda}^{\frac{1}{\lambda}}r_i^{\frac{1}{\lambda}-1}e^{-\frac{r_i}{\lambda}}\left(\frac{1}{\Gamma(1/\lambda)}\right).
\end{aligned}$$

24.6 Bernoulli Stage I and Normal Stage II

Assume we have I providers, each treating n_i patients, and let $y_{ij} = 1$ if the patient received a needed therapy and 0 otherwise. Assume $y_{ij} \mid r_i \sim \text{Bernoulli}(p_{ij})$ such that

$$\begin{aligned}
f(y_{ij}) &= p_{ij}^{y_{ij}}(1 - p_{ij})^{1-y_{ij}},\\
\log\left(\frac{p_{ij}}{1 - p_{ij}}\right) &= \mathbf{x}_{ij}\boldsymbol{\beta} + r_i.
\end{aligned}$$

If $r_i \sim N(0, \tau^2)$, then this is the generalized linear mixed model; if r_i comes from a Beta distribution, then this leads to a conjugate HGLM (using an h-likelihood).

24.6.1 Extended Likelihood

To use the extended log-likelihood,

$$\text{If } \eta_{ij} = \beta_0 + \beta_1 x_{ij} + r_i \text{ where } r_i \sim N(0, \tau^2), \text{ then}$$

$$\log f(\mathbf{y}_i) \propto \sum_{j=1}^{n_i} \Big(y_{ij}(\mathbf{x}_{ij}\boldsymbol{\beta} + r_i) - \log(1 + \exp(\mathbf{x}_{ij}\boldsymbol{\beta} + r_i)) \Big).$$

The contribution to the Stage II log-likelihood from cluster i is

$$\log g(r_i) \propto \frac{1}{2}\left(\frac{r_i^2}{\tau^2} - \log \tau^2 \right).$$

The kernel of the extended-likelihood is

$$\log h = \sum_{i=1}^{I} \sum_{j=1}^{n_i} \Big(y_{ij}(\mathbf{x}_{ij}\boldsymbol{\beta} + r_i) - \log(1 + \exp(\mathbf{x}_{ij}\boldsymbol{\beta} + r_i)) \Big) + \frac{1}{2}\left(\sum_{i=1}^{I} \frac{r_i^2}{\tau^2} - I \log \tau^2 \right).$$

24.6.2 Bayesian

A fully Bayesian approach places prior distributions on $\boldsymbol{\beta}$ and τ^2. For the regression coefficients, assume prior independence and vague Normal distributions, β_p; $p = 0, \ldots, P \sim N(0, 1000)$. An inverse Gamma distribution is used for τ^2.

24.7 Hospital Satisfaction HGLM Example

We return to the hospital satisfaction, where the outcome is now binary (see Volume 2, Chapter 21, "Hierarchical Generalized Linear Models") with a value of 1 indicating the patient was satisfied with the care received and 0 otherwise, and there are 20 hospitals. The GLLM version of the model is

$$P(Y_{ij} = 1) \sim \text{Bernoulli}(p_{ij}),$$
$$\text{logit}(p_{ij}) = \beta_0 + \beta_1 \text{Age}_{ij} + \beta_2 \text{Female}_{ij} + \beta_3 \text{Severity}_{ij} + r_i,\ r_i \sim N(0, \tau^2).$$

As in the HLM analysis of the linear satisfaction outcome, we use three different approaches for estimating the model parameters (see Box 24.6). The parameter estimates are presented in Table 24.5, and the regression coefficients are in close agreement. The between-hospital variance estimates do differ, ranging from 0.025 to 0.033. Figure 24.2 provides summaries of the between-hospital variation as well as the hospital-specific effects obtained from the Bayesian model. The posterior median of τ^2 is 0.037 compared to a posterior mean of 0.053. The posterior mean of the range in the ratio of odds ratios is 2.4 with a 95% credible interval of (1.33, 5.51). The posterior distributions of the hospital-specific effects for randomly selected 5 hospitals indicate Hospital A is shifted to the left (poorer log-odds of patient satisfaction) compared to the other hospitals. The final plot in the lower right corner of the figure presents the posterior probability that the hospital effect is smaller than −0.2, an arbitrarily selected threshold. This probability is highest in Hospital A (0.42); 3/4 of the hospitals have a probability of less than 0.24.

Box 24.6 R code for patient satisfaction via HGLM

```
Classical Likelihood
glmer(binaryy ~ (1|hosp.id) + cage + female + cseverity,data=lindata.set,
     family=binomial(link="logit"))
Extended Likelihood
hglm(fixed=binaryy ~ cage + female + cseverity,random = ~1|hosp.id,
     family=binomial(link=logit),fix.disp=1,
     rand.family=gaussian(link=identity),data=lindata.set)
Bayesian
apar=0.001; bpar=0.01
lgprior = list(prec = list(prior="loggamma",param = c(apar,bpar)))
formula = binaryy ~ cage+ female + cseverity
         + f(hosp.id,model="iid",hyper=lgprior)
inla(formula, family="binomial", data=lindata.set)
```

The Bayesian approach (INLA code) assumes the priors for $\beta_p, p = 0, 1, 2, 3$ are mutually independent, arising from $N(0, 1{,}000)$ (default), and τ^2 arise from log-gamma distribution using Gamma(0.001, 0.01).

Table 24.5 HGLM estimates (standard errors) obtained using classical likelihood, extended likelihood, and fully Bayesian approaches. Bayesian values are posterior means and posterior standard deviations.

Parameter	Likelihood-based classical	Likelihood-based extended	Posterior mean (SD)
Intercept	−2.13 (0.101)	−2.13 (0.101)	−2.15(0.110)
Age, centered	0.0401 (0.00736)	0.0400 (0.007358)	0.0403 (0.00736)
Female	−0.107(0.159)	−0.106(0.159)	−0.110(0.159)
Severity, centered	0.350 (0.0737)	0.349 (0.0736)	0.352 (0.0736)
τ^2	0.0251	0.0331	0.0525

24.8 CABG Mortality Example

Recall Example 1 introduced in Chapter 1, involving the assessment of CABG hospital surgical quality. The data include 4,603 cases treated at one of 13 Massachusetts hospitals. The total number of 30-day deaths was 101 (2.19%), with observed rates ranging from 0 to 3.94%. A fully Bayesian hierarchical logistic regression model was fitted to the data using

$$\text{logit}(P(Y_{ij} = 1 \mid \mathbf{x}_{ij}, \boldsymbol{\beta}, \alpha_i)) = \alpha_i + \mathbf{x}_{ij}\boldsymbol{\beta},$$
$$\alpha_i \sim N(\mu, \tau^2),$$
$$\mu \sim N(0, 1{,}000);\ \boldsymbol{\beta} \sim N(0, 1{,}000);\ \text{and}\ \tau^{-2} \sim \text{Gamma}(0.001, 0.001).$$

The Gamma distribution is the prior distribution for the precision, $1/\tau^2$, has a mean equal to 1, variance equal to 1,000, and is equivalent to assuming $\log(\tau^{-2})$ is uniform. The prior distributions for the regression coefficients and the mean of the

Figure 24.2 Marginal posterior densities for between-hospital variance, the range in variation, the posterior densities of r_i for five hospitals, and the posterior probability $r_i < -0.2$: patient satisfaction data. The first five hospitals in the graph in the lower right correspond to hospitals A through E.

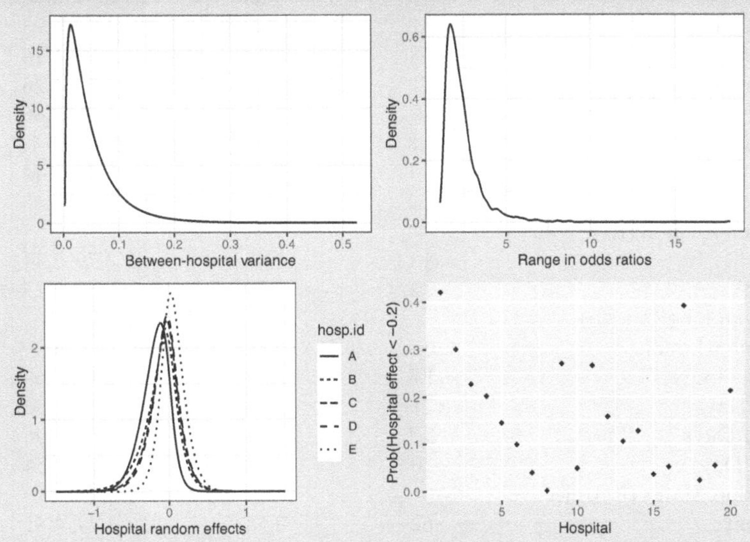

Box 24.7 Starting values hierarchical logistic regression model

Estimate the logistic regression model

$$\text{logit}\left(P(Y_{ij} = 1)\right) = b_1 + b_2 + \cdots + b_I + \mathbf{x}_{ij}\boldsymbol{\beta},$$

where b_i is the effect for hospital i after adjusting for patient risk factors. Starting values for Chain 1 are $\beta^{(0)} = \widehat{\boldsymbol{\beta}}$, $\alpha_i^{(0)} = \widehat{b}_i$, $\mu^{(0)} = \frac{1}{I}\sum_i \widehat{b}_i$, and $\tau^{2(0)} = \frac{1}{I-1}\sum_i(\widehat{b}_i - \widehat{\mu}^0)^2$. In Chain 2, an over-dispersed starting value for the variance component is selected using $\tau^{2(0)} = 10 \times \frac{1}{I-1}\sum_i(\widehat{b}_i - \widehat{\mu}^0)^2$. For Chain 3, an under-dispersed starting value for the variance component is created using $\tau^{2(0)} = 0.10 \times \frac{1}{I-1}\sum_i(\widehat{b}_i - \widehat{\mu}^0)^2$.

random effects are also non-informative. The confounders were determined a priori based on a literature review and opinions provided by clinical experts. The data source for this study was a clinical registry where items were prospectively collected and validated through an external audit. Thus, there are no missing data. The model was estimated using the Monte Carlo Markov Chain using three parallel chains. Starting values for τ^{-2} in the chains differed (see Box 24.7). Model convergence was assessed using the Gelman–Rubin statistic after a burn-in of 3,000 iterations. Inferences are based on a subsequent 3,000 iterations.

The estimated frequencies for the confounders as well as corresponding odds ratios, $\exp(\widehat{\boldsymbol{\beta}})$, estimated from the hierarchical logistic regression model are presented in Table 24.6. Three-quarters of the sample are male, 2.2% arrived in

Table 24.6 Hierarchical logistic regression (HLR) odds ratios (95% credible intervals) for 30-day mortality following CABG surgery.

Risk factor	Mean (%)	HLR odds ratio	HLR 95% interval
Years over 65	1.5	1.05	1.02, 1.07
Male	75	0.60	0.39, 0.96
Renal Failure	7.3	2.39	1.32, 3.93
Diabetes	38	1.17	0.72, 1.76
Hypertension	77	2.91	1.35, 6.26
Peripheral vascular disease	18	1.73	1.05, 2.66
Prior CABG surgery	3.8	5.83	2.83, 10.11
Prior PTCA	19	0.87	0.48, 1.44
Cardiogenic shock	2.2	3.16	1.29, 6.45
Ejection fraction (Ref: $\geqslant$ 40%)	–	–	–
< 30%	13	1.48	0.79, 2.44
30–39	12	1.33	0.68, 2.27
Heart attack (Ref: No)	–	–	–
Within 6 hours	0.9	9.89	2.44, 26.63
7 - 24 Hours	1.8	3.72	1.15, 8.68
1 - 7 Days	21	1.10	0.57, 1.90
8 - 21 Days	5.7	1.45	0.56, 2.96
> 21 Days	20	1.43	0.72, 2.54
Procedure status (Ref: elective)	–	–	–
Urgent	62	2.55	1.29, 4.81
Emergent/Salvage	3.7	2.61	1.40, 6.44
Pre-Op IABP	9.3	2.57	1.40, 4.37

PTCA, percutaneous transluminal coronary angioplasty; IABP, intra-aortic balloon pump.

cardiogenic shock, and 62% of the surgeries are classified as urgent. Cardiogenic shock and having a heart attack within 24 hours of the surgery increase mortality substantially. Pre-operative intra-aortic balloon pump use was included in the model, as the national STS model had included it. In retrospect, this variable should be excluded, as it is a practice style and potentially on the causal pathway of the effect of hospital quality on mortality.[6]

The estimate of the between-hospital standard deviation, on the logit scale, is 0.205. Thus, a patient undergoing surgery at a high-mortality hospital (defined as 1 standard deviation above the mean) is 1.5 times as likely to die within 30 days of CABG surgery compared to a patient treated at a low-mortality hospital (defined as 1 standard deviation below the mean), a meaningful difference.

To assess hospital performance, the standardized mortality incidence rate (SMIR) is estimated for each hospital. The typical approach fits a logistic regression to the outcome, obtains parameter estimates for the coefficients, $\widehat{\gamma}$, and using these estimates, determines the number of deaths at each hospital given the hospital's case-mix by summing over the predicted probabilities of death for patients in the hospital, for example, $\sum_j \text{logit}^{-1}(\widehat{\gamma}_0 + \mathbf{x}_{ij}\widehat{\boldsymbol{\gamma}})$. The observed number

[6] Models in subsequent years excluded pre-op IABP.

Figure 24.3 Standardized mortality incident rates following CABG surgery. Upper points correspond to estimates using a logistic regression model, U_i; lower points are posterior means from the hierarchical logistic regression model, S_i. Dashed vertical line is the state-observed rate. Numbers below the upper x-axis are the number of cases in each hospital.

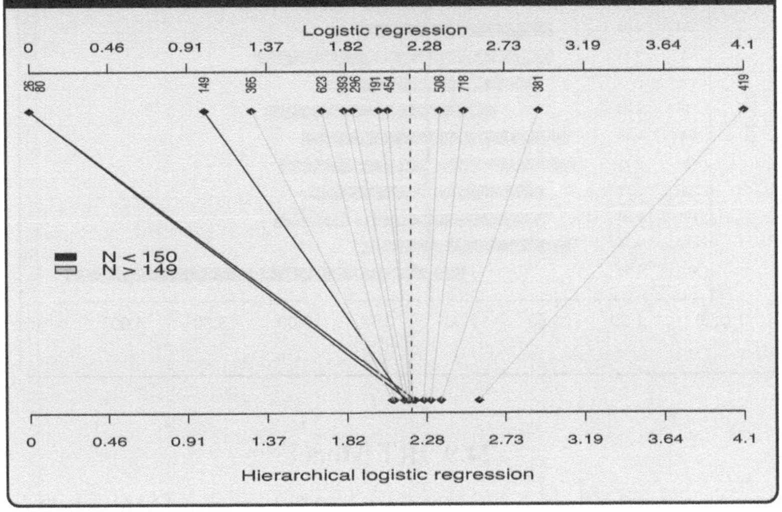

of deaths is then compared to the expected number of deaths by creating a ratio of the two. Hospital-specific estimates using the hierarchical model, S_i, and the usual approach, U_i, are defined as

$$S_i = \frac{\sum_{j=1}^{n_j} \text{logit}^{-1}(\widehat{\alpha}_i + \mathbf{x}_{ij}\widehat{\boldsymbol{\beta}})}{\sum_{j=1}^{n_i} \text{logit}^{-1}(\widehat{\mu} + \mathbf{x}_{ij}\widehat{\boldsymbol{\beta}})} \times \bar{y} \text{ and } U_i = \frac{\sum_{j=1}^{n_j} y_{ij}}{\sum_{j=1}^{n_i} \text{logit}^{-1}(\widehat{\gamma}_0 + \mathbf{x}_{ij}\widehat{\boldsymbol{\gamma}})} \times \bar{y}$$

$$\text{where } \bar{y} = \frac{1}{\sum_i n_i} \sum_{i,j} y_{ij}. \tag{24.25}$$

The values, U_i,[7] are plotted against the hierarchical regression estimates, S_i, in Figure 24.3. The U_i's are shrunk toward the overall mean (dashed vertical line) at $\bar{y} = 2.19\%$, with smaller volume hospital estimates, as expected, shrinking more, although all estimates change. The range in the SMIRs based on U_is is much smaller than the range of those based on S_i.

The hospital with the highest estimated SMIR is the same whether using U_i or S_i. The two hospitals having 0 deaths have $U_i = 0$ but using the hierarchical model, these hospitals no longer have the smallest value of the S_i. Figure 24.4 displays the S_is and corresponding 95% credible intervals. The hospital with 419 cases has an SMIR of 2.58 with a 95% interval shifted to the right relative to any other hospital. This hospital had 15 30-day deaths (3.58%); the largest unadjusted hospital percentage was 3.94, also corresponding to 15 observed deaths.

[7] These are taken from Example 1, in Volume 1, Chapter 2, "Conceptual Models."

Figure 24.4 Standardized mortality incident rates following CABG surgery.

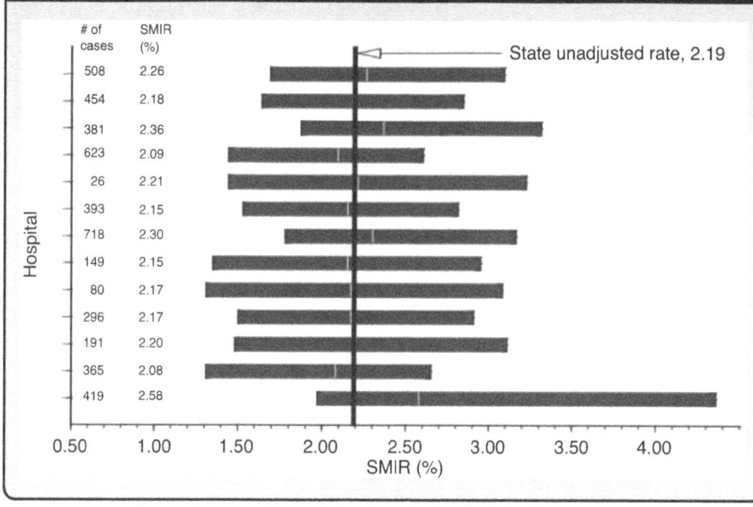

24.9 IRT Model

Recall from Volume 2, Chapter 22, "Composite Measures and Multiple Outcomes," the 2-parameter logistic model for a binary response, Y_{ij}, by person i for item j is defined as

$$p_{ij} = P(Y_{ij} = 1 \mid \theta_i) = \frac{\exp(a_j(\theta_i - b_j))}{1 + \exp(a_j(\theta_i - b_j))}; \quad a_j > 0,$$

and, without loss of generality, assume $Y_{ij} = 1$ denotes better quality of care compared to $Y_{ij} = 0$. In the model, θ_j is the underlying latent trait, a_j is the item discrimination parameter assumed to be positive so that persons with $Y_{ij} = 1$ have better quality of care than persons with $Y_{ij} = 0$, and b_j is an item difficulty parameter. The larger the value of a_j, the more discriminating item j is. Assuming $i = 1, \ldots, n$ persons, and $j = 1, \ldots, J$ items, the likelihood of the data is given by

$$\prod_{i=1}^{n} \phi(\theta_i) \prod_{j=1}^{J} p_{ij}^{y_{ij}} (1 - p_{ij})^{1-y_{ij}}.$$

It is assumed $\theta_i \sim N(0, 1)$. In the model,there are $n + 2J$ unknown parameters, $\boldsymbol{\theta} = (\theta_1, \theta_2, \ldots, \theta_n)$, $\boldsymbol{\zeta}_j = (a_j, b_j)$. If the θ_i are considered nuisance parameters, then the marginal likelihood is given by

$$p(\boldsymbol{\zeta} \mid \mathbf{Y}) = \int_{\boldsymbol{\theta}} p(\boldsymbol{\theta}, \boldsymbol{\zeta} \mid \mathbf{Y}) d\boldsymbol{\theta},$$

so that the number of unknown parameters is now $2I$. The logarithm of the marginal likelihood is

$$L(\boldsymbol{\zeta} \mid \mathbf{Y}) = \sum_{i=1}^{n} \log \left(\int_{\theta_i} \phi(\theta_i) \prod_{j=1}^{J} p_{ij}^{y_{ij}} (1 - p_{ij})^{1-y_{ij}} d\theta_i \right).$$

24.9.1 Extended Likelihood

Using Newton–Raphson, differentiating the marginal log-likelihood with respect to a_j and b_j yields[8]

$$\sum_{i=1}^{n} Y_{ij} = \sum_{i=1}^{n} \int_{\theta_i} \frac{\exp(a_j\theta_i - b_j^*)p(\theta_i \mid \mathbf{Y}, \boldsymbol{\zeta})}{1+\exp(a_j\theta_i - b_j^*)} d\theta_i,$$

$$\sum_{j=1}^{n} Y_{ij} \int_{\theta_i} p(\theta_i \mid \mathbf{Y}, \boldsymbol{\zeta}) d\theta_i = \sum_{i=1}^{n} \int_{\theta_i} \frac{\exp(a_j\theta_i - b_j^*)p(\theta_i \mid \mathbf{Y}, \boldsymbol{\zeta})}{1+\exp(a_j\theta_i - b_j^*)} d\theta_i$$

for $j = 1, \ldots, J$ and where $p(\theta_i \mid \mathbf{Y}, \boldsymbol{\zeta})$ is proportional to $\phi(\theta_i) \prod_{j=1}^{J} p_{ij}^{y_{ij}} (1-p_{ij})^{1-y_{ij}}$. These equations must be solved numerically.

24.9.2 Bayesian

A Bayesian approach introduces a latent variable $Z_{ij} \sim N(a_j(\theta_i - b_j), 1)$ where $Y_{ij} = 1$ if $Z_{ij} > 0$; otherwise $Y_{ij} = 0$. Let $\mathbf{Z} = (Z_{11}, Z_{12}, \ldots, Z_{nJ})$; $\boldsymbol{\zeta}_j = (a_j, b_j^*)$ and $\boldsymbol{\zeta} = (\xi_1, \xi_2, \ldots, \xi_J)$; and $\boldsymbol{\theta} = (\theta_1, \theta_2, \ldots, \theta_n)$. Prior distributions are required for the components of $\boldsymbol{\zeta}_j$ which we take to be non-informative with

$$\pi(\boldsymbol{\zeta}_j) = \pi(a_j)\pi(b_j^*) \propto \prod_{j=1}^{J} I(a_j > 0),$$

where we have assumed a priori independence between a_j and b_j. Gibbs sampling is utilized, and so we require the full conditional distributions for $\boldsymbol{\zeta}$, θ_i, and $\mathbf{Z}$. These are

$$Z_{ij} \mid \boldsymbol{\theta}, \boldsymbol{\zeta}, \mathbf{Y} \sim \begin{cases} N(a_j\theta_i - b_j^*, 1) \text{ truncated at the left by 0 if } Y_{ij} = 1, \\ N(a_j\theta_i - b_j^*, 1) \text{ truncated at the right by 0 if } Y_{ij} = 0, \end{cases}$$

$$\theta_i \mid \mathbf{Z}, \boldsymbol{\zeta} \sim N\left(\frac{\widehat{\theta_i}}{1+A}, \frac{A}{1+A}\right), \; A = \left\{\sum_{j=1}^{J} a_j^2\right\}^{-1}, \text{ and } \widehat{\theta_i} = A \sum_{j=1}^{J} a_j(Z_{ij} + b_j^*),$$

$$\boldsymbol{\zeta}_j \mid \boldsymbol{\theta}, \mathbf{Z} \sim N_2((H^\top H)^{-1} H^\top \mathbf{Z}_j, (H^\top H)^{-1}) \text{ for } a_j > 0, \text{ where}$$

$$H = \begin{pmatrix} \theta_1 & -1 \\ \theta_2 & -1 \\ \vdots & \vdots \\ \theta_n & -1 \end{pmatrix} \text{ and } \mathbf{Z}_j = \begin{pmatrix} Z_{1j} \\ Z_{2j} \\ \vdots \\ Z_{nj} \end{pmatrix}.$$

Now, suppose we associate each person with a medical provider indexed by $k = 1, \ldots, K$, and each provider is associated with n_k person. The model becomes

$$P(Y_{kij} = 1 \mid \theta_{ki}) = \frac{\exp(a_j\theta_{ki} - b_j^*)}{1+\exp(a_j\theta_{ki} - b_j^*)} \tag{24.26}$$

[8] $b_j^* = a_j b_j$.

where only the latent trait, θ_{ki}, is indexed by provider. The structural model links the latent trait to person characteristics such that the associations are permitted to vary across providers

$$\theta_{ki} = \mathbf{X}_{ki}^{\top}\boldsymbol{\gamma}_k + \delta_{ki},\ \delta_{ki} \sim N(0, \sigma^2) \tag{24.27}$$

noting that $\mathbf{X}_{ki}$ is a $1 \times p$ vector containing person characteristics and an intercept term. The term δ_{ki} reflects residual variation in quality provided to an individual not accounted for by covariates. To accommodate variation between providers,

$$\boldsymbol{\gamma}_k = \boldsymbol{\mu} + \boldsymbol{\epsilon}_k \quad \boldsymbol{\epsilon}_k \sim N_p(\mathbf{0}, T). \tag{24.28}$$

Non-informative prior distributions will be assumed for $\boldsymbol{\zeta}_j$, σ^2, $\boldsymbol{\mu}$, and T. An improper non-informative prior μ is assumed,

$$\pi(\boldsymbol{\mu}) = \ \propto c.$$

For the variance components, non-informative priors are

$$\pi(\sigma^2) \propto \sigma^{-2} \ \& \ \pi(T) \propto T^{-1}.$$

The full conditionals for Z_{kij} are similar to the model without the provider effect,

$$Z_{kij} \mid \boldsymbol{\theta}, \boldsymbol{\zeta}, \mathbf{Y} \sim \begin{cases} N(a_j\theta_{ki} - b_j^*, 1) \text{ truncated at the left by 0 if } Y_{kij} = 1, \\ N(a_j\theta_{ki} - b_j^*, 1) \text{ truncated at the right by 0 if } Y_{kij} = 0. \end{cases}$$

The quality parameter is now a function of the item parameters and person-specific covariates,

$$\theta_{ki} \mid Z_{kij}, \boldsymbol{\zeta}, \boldsymbol{\gamma}_k, \sigma^2 \sim N\left(\frac{A\widehat{\theta}_{ki} + \sigma^{-2}\mathbf{X}_{ki}^{\top}\boldsymbol{\gamma}_k}{A + \sigma^{-2}}, \frac{1}{A + \sigma^{-2}}\right), \ \widehat{\theta}_{ki} = A\sum_{j=1}^{J} a_j(Z_{kij} + b_j^*),$$
$$\text{and } A = \left\{\sum_{j=1}^{J} a_j^2\right\}^{-1}.$$

The full conditional for the item parameters is the same as before with

$$\boldsymbol{\zeta}_j \mid \boldsymbol{\theta}, \mathbf{Z}_j \sim N_2((H^{\top}H)^{-1}H^{\top}\mathbf{Z}_j, (H^{\top}H)^{-1}) \text{ for } a_j > 0.$$

The provider-specific regression coefficient arises from a multivariate Normal

$$\boldsymbol{\gamma}_k \mid \boldsymbol{\theta}_k, \sigma^2, \boldsymbol{\mu}, T \sim N_p(Bb, B),\ \Sigma_k^{-1} = \sigma^2(\mathbf{X}_k^{\top}\mathbf{X}_k)^{-1},\ B = (\Sigma_k^{-1} + T^{-1})^{-1},$$
$$\text{and } b = \Sigma_k^{-1}\widehat{\boldsymbol{\gamma}}_k + T^{-1}\boldsymbol{\mu}$$

where $\widehat{\gamma}_k = (\mathbf{X}_k^{\top}\mathbf{X}_k)^{-1}\mathbf{X}_k^{\top}\boldsymbol{\theta}_k$. Thus, the mean is a weighted sum of the least squares estimator and the prior mean. Next,

$$\boldsymbol{\mu} \mid \boldsymbol{\gamma}_k, T \sim N_2\left(\frac{1}{K}\sum_{k=1}^{K}\boldsymbol{\gamma}_k, \frac{1}{K}T\right),$$

which, unsurprisingly, is the average of the provider-specific parameters. Letting $N = \sum_{k=1}^{K} n_k$, then

$$\sigma^2 \mid \boldsymbol{\theta}, \boldsymbol{\gamma} \sim \text{Inv-}\chi^2\left(N, \frac{1}{N}\sum_{k=1}^{K}(\boldsymbol{\theta}_k - \mathbf{X}_k^\top \boldsymbol{\gamma}_k)^\top(\boldsymbol{\theta}_k - \mathbf{X}_k^\top \boldsymbol{\gamma}_k)\right) \text{ and}$$

$$T \mid \boldsymbol{\gamma}_k, \boldsymbol{\mu} \sim \text{Inv-Wishart}\left(\sum_{k=1}^{K}(\boldsymbol{\gamma}_k - \boldsymbol{\mu})(\boldsymbol{\gamma}_k - \boldsymbol{\mu})^\top, K\right).$$

24.10 Summary

Inferences for HGLMs may be based on the extended log-likelihood approach or a Bayesian approach. The two approaches differ fundamentally in terms of the interpretation of probability. This fundamental difference is important when interpreting findings. Beyond that, both approaches (1) assume independence of observations within clusters conditional on random effects and (2) specify a probability distribution for the random effects. The extended likelihood imposes a constraint on the mean of the random effects, whereas in the Bayesian approach, prior distributions for the parameters governing the random effect distributions are specified. Within the extended likelihood framework, maximizing the joint likelihood of the fixed and random effects provides valid inferences if the random effects appear linearly in the linear predictor scale. The Bayesian approach does not restrict the scale of the random effects, although computational complexity increases with non-conjugate prior distributions. A compelling feature of the Bayesian approach is the ease with which to compute estimates of functions of the parameters and their associated measures of uncertainty—each drawn from the joint posterior distribution is used to form the distribution for the function of interest. Outside the Bayesian framework, bootstrapping methods can be used to resample units repeatedly.

CHAPTER TWENTY-FIVE

Model Assessment

Assumptions associated with the HGLM were described in Volume 2, Chapters 20 and 21. These include conditional independence, distributional assumptions for each level of the hierarchy, functional form of the covariates, exchangeability (if adopting a Bayesian framework), and independence of the random effects with the person-level covariates. In this chapter, we describe how to use the error components defined at each level of the hierarchy to check the validity of the assumptions made. Model selection, that is, which model from a set of models should be used, uses global measures to minimize overall model error subject to the number of model parameters. We discuss various global measures, noting that the choice of measure depends upon whether the models considered are nested or not. A key metric in generalized linear models is the deviance, which we will also exploit. If adopting a Bayesian approach, a comparison of replicated data generated from the posterior distribution can be used to assess the appropriateness of model assumptions. We describe this approach, denoted posterior predictive checks, which ends up being a powerful tool. Finally, we describe approaches to assessing the validity of causal inference assumptions.

25.1 Error Components

Let $y_{11}, y_{12}, \ldots, y_{In_i}$ denote the observed data and adopt the generalized linear mixed model formulation of the HGLM, where $\mathbf{z}_{ij} \in \mathbf{x}_{ij}$ and

1. Stage I. Conditional on the random effects, r_i, the outcomes are independent and arise from a GLM, where $\mathbb{E}(y_{ij} \mid \mathbf{r}_i) = \mu_{ij}$, $\text{Var}(y_{ij} \mid \mathbf{r}_i) = \phi V(\mu_{ij})$, $\eta_{ij} = l(\mu_{ij}) = \mathbf{x}_{ij}\boldsymbol{\beta} + \mathbf{z}_{ij}\boldsymbol{\nu}_i$, and $\boldsymbol{\nu}_i = \nu(\mathbf{r}_i)$.
2. Stage II. The random effects are independent and identically distributed from a one parameter exponential with $\mathbb{E}(r_i) = \psi_R$, and $\text{Var}(r_i) = \rho \text{V}(\psi_R)$.

where $\mathbb{E}(r_i)$ is constrained such that $\nu(r_i) = 0$. Denote $\widehat{\beta}$ as the estimate for the fixed effects and $\widehat{\nu_i}$ as the estimate for the random effects.

1. $\widehat{e_{ij}} = y_{ij} - \mathbf{x}_{ij}\widehat{\boldsymbol{\beta}} - \mathbf{z}_i\widehat{\nu_i}$ is the residual for $\mathbb{E}(Y_{ij} \mid \mathbf{r}_i)$.
   (a) Plot $\widehat{e_{ij}}$ against $g^{-1}(\mathbf{x}_{ij}\widehat{\beta})$. No systematic pattern should be apparent.
   (b) Plot $|\widehat{e_{ij}}|$ against $g^{-1}(\mathbf{x}_{ij}\widehat{\beta})$. No systematic pattern should be apparent.

Figure 25.1 Estimates from the HLM of patient satisfaction data. (a) Studentized and (b) | Studentized| residuals against fitted values; (c) Q–Q plot of residuals; and (d) histogram of residuals.

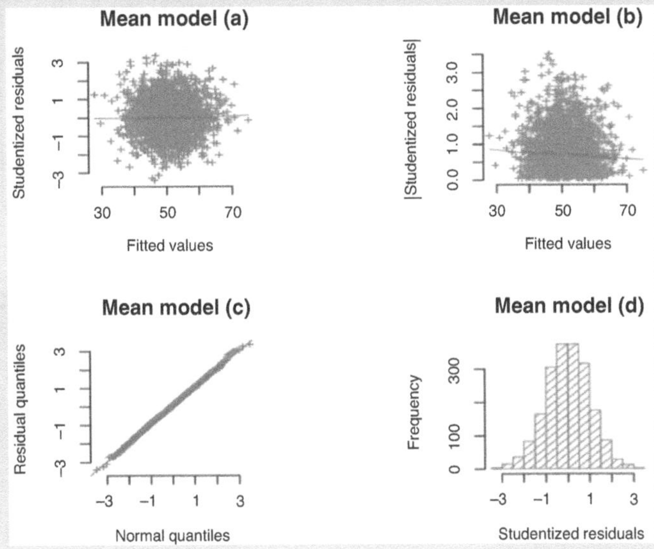

2. If there is any temporal ordering to the data, plot the residuals against time. Any systematic pattern may indicate serial or temporal dependence.
3. Construct histograms of the residuals. The distribution should be symmetric around 0.

Figure 25.1 displays the residuals from the patient satisfaction data using the HLM described in Volume 2, Chapter 24, "Inference for Hierarchical Generalized Linear Models." The model fits well as no pattern is identified in figures (a) and (b); the residuals are centered on 0 (d) and the normality assumption appears fine (c).

25.2 Comparing Models

25.2.1 Deviance

Suppose there are two competing models, M_1 and M_2, and the goal is to determine which model fits the data better. Several measures are available to compare models, although some measures require that the models are nested (one model is a submodel of the other model), while others do not. The deviance is a measure of goodness-of-fit defined as a linear function of the log-likelihood,

$$D = -2\left\{l(\widehat{\mu}, y) - l(y, y)\right\}, \tag{25.1}$$

where $l(\widehat{\mu}, y)$ is the log-likelihood evaluated at the maximum likelihood estimator $\widehat{\mu}$, and $l(y, y)$ is the log-likelihood for an exact fit. $l(y, y)$ denotes the full model

Table 25.1 Deviance functions for GLMS. Note that $\mathbb{E}(y_{ij}) = \mu_{ij}$; n_{ij} is the denominator for the Binomial distribution.

$Y_{ij} \mid r_i$ Distribution	Deviance, D
Normal	$(y_{ij} - \widehat{\mu}_{ij})^2$
Poisson	$2\{y_{ij}\log(y_{ij}/\widehat{\mu}_{ij}) - (y_{ij} - \widehat{\mu}_{ij})^2\}$
Binomial	$2\left\{y_{ij}\log(y_{ij}/\widehat{\mu}_{ij}) + (n_{ij} - y_{ij})\log\left(\frac{n_{ij}-y_{ij}}{n_{ij}-\widehat{\mu}_{ij}}\right)\right\}$
Gamma	$2\{-\log(y_{ij}/\widehat{\mu}_{ij}) + (y_{ij} - \widehat{\mu}_{ij}/\widehat{\mu}_{ij}\}$
Beta	$2\left\{\widehat{\mu}_{ij}\log(\widehat{\mu}_{ij}/y_{ij}) + (n_{ji} - \widehat{\mu}_{ij})\log\left(\frac{n_{ij}-\widehat{\mu}_{ij}}{n_{ij}-ryij}\right)\right\}$

Box 25.1 Number of parameters (model complexity)

In a generalized linear model with p covariates, the number of parameters is p. In a HGLM described by $\mathbb{E}(Y_{ij}) = l^{-1}(\mu_{ij})$ with $l(\mu_{ij}) = \mathbf{x}_{ij}\boldsymbol{\beta} + \mathbf{z}_{ij}v(\mathbf{r}_i)$, $\text{Var}(Y_{ij}) = \phi V(\mu_{ij})$, $\mathbb{E}(r_i) = \psi_R$, and $\text{Var}(r_i) = \rho V(\psi_R)$, the number of parameters is

$$p_D = \text{trace}\{(T^\top \Sigma^{-1} T)^{-1}(T^\top \Sigma_w^{-1} T)\}$$

$$\text{where } T = \begin{pmatrix} X & Z \\ 0 & I \end{pmatrix};\ \Sigma_w^{-1} = W\{\text{diag}(\boldsymbol{\phi}^{-1}, 0)\} \text{ and } W = \text{diag}(W_y, W_r)$$

where $W_y = \left(\frac{\partial \mu_i}{\partial \eta_i}\right)^2 V(\mu_i)^{-1}$, $W_r = \left(\frac{\partial r_i}{\partial v_i}\right)^2 V(r_i)^{-1}$ and Σ is defined below Eq. (24.17).

and lies at the extreme, as there is no summary of the data. The deviance is additive for nested sets of models. Table 25.1 describes the deviance functions for some exponential families.

When observations are independent, then

$$D = \sum_i \sum_j d_{ij},$$

where d_{ij} represents the contribution to the deviance for the jth observation in the ith cluster. Noting that $\mathbb{E}(D) \approx n - p_D$, where p_D is a measure of the number of parameters (Box 25.1), the Deviance Information Criterion (DIC) is a scaled deviance defined as

$$DIC = D + 2p_D. \tag{25.2}$$

The goal is to choose the model that minimizes the DIC. There is no requirement that the models be nested. To compare two nested models, the difference in the two deviances,

$$DIC_1 - DIC_2. \tag{25.3}$$

Differences of more than 10 between two models rule out the model with the higher DIC, differences between 5 and 10 are substantial, and differences less than 5 may not be meaningful. The DIC has been criticized for selecting overly complex models.

For HGLM, Lee and Nelder [79] suggest using three different measures of deviance for testing the model components (random, fixed, and dispersion) of the hierarchical model. For testing random effects, they suggest using the conditional log-likelihood; for fixed coefficients, the marginal log-likelihood; and for the dispersion parameters, the REML log-likelihood.

25.2.2 Cross-Validation

A common approach to assessing model fit involves setting aside a portion of the data for validation purposes, with the majority of the sample used to develop the model. The approach assumes that the "true" model generates better out-of-sample predictions than a competing model. Once the model is finalized, the fit of the model is assessed using the validation sample. If the sample size is too small to set aside a validation sample, a cross-validation approach can be adopted. The cross-validated residual is defined as

$$\widehat{e}^*_{ij} = y_{ij} - E(Y_{ij} \mid r_i, \mathbf{Y}_{i,-j}),$$

where the notation $\mathbf{Y}_{i,-j}$ denotes all the data excluding observation Y_{ij}. Large values suggest Y_{ij} is influential. Entire clusters could also be eliminated to detect if some clusters are influential. Cross-validation is a simple and intuitive approach that is broadly applicable.

25.3 Bayesian-Specific Procedures

25.3.1 Conditional Predictive Ordinate

Related to cross-validation, the conditional predictive ordinate (CPO) is the value of posterior predictive density at the value $Y_{ij} = y_{ij}$, when the predictive density is from all the data points except for the ijth point, for example,

$$f(Y_{ij} \mid \mathbf{Y}_{i,-j} = \int f(Y_{ij} \mid \boldsymbol{\theta}, Y_{i,-j})\pi(\boldsymbol{\theta} \mid Y_{i,-j})d\boldsymbol{\theta}.$$

Small values of CPO indicate poor model fit.

25.3.2 Replication and Bayesian p-Value

The basic idea is to define a test quantity, which is a scalar summary of parameters and data, and then examine the tail-area probability of the test quantity. The posterior predictive distribution is defined as

$$f(y^{\text{rep}} \mid \mathbf{y}) = \int f(y^{\text{rep}} \mid \theta)p(\theta \mid \mathbf{y})d\theta,$$

where y^{rep} refers to replicated data and $\mathbf{y}$ refers to the observed data. y^{rep} is specifically a replication like y. Let $T(y, \theta)$ represent the discrepancy measure. The classical p-value for the test statistic, $T(y)$, is

$$Pr(T(y^{\text{rep}}) \geqslant T(y) \mid \theta),$$

where the probability is taken over the distribution of y^{rep} with θ fixed at $\widehat{\theta}$. In contrast, the *posterior predictive p-value* for a test statistic, $T(y, \theta)$, is defined as

$$Pr(T(y^{\text{rep}}, \theta) \geqslant T(y, \theta) \mid \mathbf{y}),$$

which is calculated as

$$\int_{y^{\text{rep}}} \int_{\theta} I_{T(y^{\text{rep}}, \theta) \geqslant T(y, \theta)} p(\theta \mid \mathbf{y}) f(y^{\text{rep}} \mid \theta) d\theta dy^{\text{rep}}.$$

How to select values for $T(y, \theta)$ for assessing model fit? A good strategy is to select quantities that measure features of the data that are not directly addressed by the probability model. For instance, ranks of the sample (e.g., the minimum y), correlation of model residuals with an explanatory variable, or the χ^2 discrepancy measure

$$\sum_{ij} \frac{(y_{ij} - E(y_{ij} \mid \theta))^2}{\text{Var}(y_{ij} \mid \theta)}.$$

Large values (close to 1) or small values (close to 0) indicate the model is suspect. The Bayesian P-value should not be compared across different models. The Bayesian P-value is **not** the probability that the model is correct. It provides information about model adequacy. One potential limitation is that the data used are twice (once to compute the observed statistic and again to compute the posterior predictive distribution). If the sample is sufficiently large, it could split into a validation and fitting sample.

25.3.3 Example 1: Hospital Mortality Following CABG Surgery

Example 1 involved assessing surgical quality for 13 Massachusetts hospitals treating 4,603 adults undergoing CABG surgery. Recall the model estimated (see Volume 2, Chapter 24, "Inference for Hierarchical Generalized Linear Models") was

$$\begin{aligned}
\text{logit}(P(Y_{ij} = 1 \mid \mathbf{x}_{ij}, \boldsymbol{\beta}, \alpha_i)) &= \alpha_i + \mathbf{x}_i \boldsymbol{\beta}, \\
\alpha_i &\sim N(\mu, \tau^2), \\
\mu &\sim N(0, 1000);\ \boldsymbol{\beta} \sim N(0, 1000);\ \text{and} \\
\tau^{-2} &\sim \text{Gamma}(0.001, 0.001).
\end{aligned}$$

Referring to Figure 24.4, from Volume 2, Chapter 24, "Inference for Hierarchical Generalized Linear Models," the wide credible interval associated with Hospital 13 may be surprising given the large sample size ($n_{13} = 419$) associated with this hospital. Does this indicate a problem with model? Figure 25.2 presents the hospital-specific estimates, $\widehat{\alpha}_i$, the numerator and denominator of the SMIRs, and the SMIRs for each hospital. Relative to the hospital-specific estimate, the expected mortality risk at Hospital 13 is much smaller, leading to larger SMIR values compared to the other hospitals.

Table 25.2 presents the posterior predictive P-values when predicting the number of deaths at each hospital i using information from all other hospitals. The posterior means of the Stage II parameters are also reported. The P-value for Hospital 13 is small, suggesting that this hospital is unusual compared to the other hospitals.

Figure 25.2 Estimates from the hierarchical logistic regression model. (a) Graph displays $\widehat{\alpha}_i$; (b) displays $\sum_{j=1}^{n_j} \text{logit}^{-1}(\widehat{\alpha}_i + \mathbf{x}_{ij}\widehat{\boldsymbol{\beta}})/n_i$; (c) $\sum_{j=1}^{n_j} \text{logit}^{-1}(\widehat{\mu} + \mathbf{x}_{ij}\widehat{\boldsymbol{\beta}})/n_i$; and (d) displays the SMIRs.

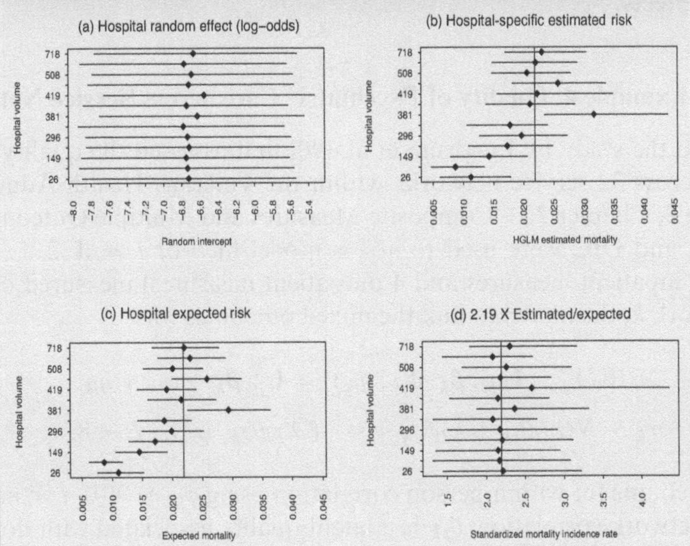

Table 25.2 Cross-validation for identifying outlying hospitals

Hospital	Volume	Posterior predictive p-value	μ_{-i}	τ^2_{-i}
1	508	0.40	−6.46	$(0.174)^2$
2	454	0.49	−6.73	$(0.183)^2$
3	381	0.12	−6.82	$(0.182)^2$
4	623	0.22	−7.19	$(0.185)^2$
5	26	0.26	−6.53	$(0.158)^2$
6	393	0.30	−6.95	$(0.180)^2$
7	718	0.33	−6.96	$(0.187)^2$
8	149	0.35	−6.77	$(0.137)^2$
9	80	0.47	−6.48	$(0.149)^2$
10	296	0.45	−6.60	$(0.199)^2$
11	191	0.43	−6.57	$(0.184)^2$
12	365	0.17	−6.69	$(0.160)^2$
13	419	0.01	−6.54	$(0.127)^2$
All hospitals	4603	–	−6.75	$(0.205)^2$

Examination of the between-hospital variance component (on logit scale) indicates that the between-hospital standard deviation with Hospital 13 removed is 3/5ths that of when it is included. Does this mean the model does not fit? One may be tempted to change the model to accommodate the additional variability introduced by Hospital 13. This could be achieved by using a t-distribution for the random effects rather than a normal distribution to permit thicker tails. However, in assessing provider quality, it is important to keep in mind that the goal is not to have the model fit well per se; rather, the goal is to determine whether particular providers are far from the "norm." Hospital 13 does appear to be far in the tail of the distribution of hospital effects.

25.3.4 Example 4: Quality of Psychiatric Care across Service Networks

Returning to the study by Landrum et al. [90] that assessed the quality of psychiatric care across 22 service networks within the Veterans Health Administration (see Volume 2, Chapter 22, "Composite Measures and Multiple Outcomes"), sample splitting and DIC were used to assess model fit. For $i = 1, 2, \ldots, 8$ quality measures (4 inpatient measures and 4 outpatient measures) measured on patient j within network k, the model to link the mixed outcomes was

$$l_k(\mathbb{E}(Y^*_{ijk} \mid \mathbf{U}_{ijk}, \boldsymbol{\beta}_k, \phi_{jk}, \eta_{ik})) = \mathbf{U}^\top_{ijk}\boldsymbol{\beta}_k + \phi_{jk} + \eta_{ik},$$
$$\eta_{ik} \sim N(\lambda_{1i}\theta_{1k} + \lambda_{2i}\theta_{2k} + \cdots + \lambda_{Li}\theta_{Lk}, \psi_i^2), \quad L < 8,$$

where ϕ_{jk} accounts for within-person correlation using $\phi_{jk} \sim N(0, \tau^2)$; η_{ik} accounts for within-network correlation; θ_{pk} is a latent quality associated with domain p for network k; λ_{1i} is a factor loading; and L is the number of latent constructs. With a sample size of about 38,000, the authors split the sample in half, one a developmental sample and the other a validation sample. To assess model fit, the authors assumed $L = 1, 2,$ and 3 latent factors and compared the models using the DIC (Table 25.3).

The DIC favors a one latent construct model, although the values across the three different models are close. The authors also used replication and posterior predictive p-values. They generated "replicated" outcomes for patients having characteristics observed in the validation using parameters from the posterior distribution determined from the developmental sample. They reported the fraction of times the pairwise correlations of the metrics at the network level in the replicated

Table 25.3 Deviance information criterion for service network example. DIC uses 100 iterations drawn from the posterior distribution.

Number of latent factors, L	DIC
One	215,568
Two	215,621
Three	215,616

sample were more extreme than the correlations observed in the validation sample, for example,

$$T(y^{rep}, \Omega) = \text{cor}(\bar{y}^{rep}_{i,\cdot k}, \bar{y}^{rep}_{i*\cdot k})\ i \neq i*,$$

where Ω contains all the parameters estimated using the developmental sample. With eight measures, there are 28 pairwise correlations. The one-, two-, and three-latent construct models had posterior p-values < 0.05 in 6/28, 6/28, and 5/28, suggesting all models were able to capture the majority of the relationships at the network level.[1] The authors selected the model with $L = 2$ because the DIC and posterior predictive checks did not really favor one model, and prior opinion indicated two latent traits (one inpatient and one ambulatory).

25.3.5 Bayes Factors

A Bayes factor is a quantity used to test hypotheses in the Bayesian framework but also can be used to compare models (see Jeffreys [126], Kass and Raftery [127]). Suppose there are two competing models, M_s. The marginal distribution for the data is

$$p(\mathbf{y} \mid M_s) = \int f(\mathbf{y} \mid \boldsymbol{\theta}_s, M_s) p(\boldsymbol{\theta}_s) d\boldsymbol{\theta}_s,\ s = 1, 2.$$

The Bayes factor in **favor** of M_1 is defined as the posterior to prior odds of M_1 divided by the posterior to prior odds of M_2:

$$BF = \frac{p(M_1 \mid \mathbf{y})/p(M_1)}{p(M_2 \mid \mathbf{y})/p(M_2)} = \frac{\left(\frac{p(M_1 \mid \mathbf{y})}{p(M_2 \mid \mathbf{y})}\right)}{\left(\frac{p(M_1)}{p(M_2)}\right)}. \tag{25.4}$$

By Bayes theorem,

$$p(M_1 \mid \mathbf{y}) = \frac{f(\mathbf{y} \mid M_1)\, p(M_1)}{f(\mathbf{y} \mid M_1) p(M_1) + f(\mathbf{y} \mid M_2) p(M_2)}.$$

Substituting these into the equation above yields the Bayes factor in favour of M_1

$$BF = \frac{f(\mathbf{y} \mid M_1)}{f(\mathbf{y} \mid M_2)}. \tag{25.5}$$

Large values of BF favor M_1 (Table 25.4).

Computation of Bayes factors can be demanding, requiring simulation or approximations [128]. On the positive side, the Bayes factor does not require models to be nested and has the attractive interpretation of a posterior to prior odds ratio. It reduces to the likelihood ratio test in the case of a simple versus simple hypothesis test. However, the Bayes factor is defined only when proper prior distributions are defined for θ. It is also sensitive to the choice of prior distributions or the choice of priors for hyperparameters. For example, if $\theta_i \sim N(\mu_0, \tau_0^2)$, the Bayes factor may become sensitive as $\tau_0^2 \to \infty$.

[1] All posterior p-values were >0.05 when examining the pairwise correlations in the validation data.

Table 25.4a Strength of evidence for interpreting Bayes factors: Jeffreys [126]

$log_{10}(BF)$	Bayes factor (BF)	
0–0.5	$1 \leqslant BF \leqslant 3.2$	Weak
0.5–1.0	$3.2 < BF \leqslant 10$	Substantial
1.0–2.0	$10 < BF \leqslant 100$	Strong
>2.0	$BF > 100$	Decisive

Table 25.4b Strength of evidence for interpreting Bayes factors: Kass and Raftery [127]

$2log(BF)$	Bayes factor (BF)	
0–2	$1 \leqslant BF \leqslant 3$	Weak
2–6	$3 < BF \leqslant 20$	Positive
6–10	$20 < BF \leqslant 150$	Strong
>10	$BF > 150$	Very strong

25.3.6 Model Averaging

A different approach averages findings over several plausible models rather than selecting a "best" model. Suppose the candidate models are $(M_1, M_2, \ldots, M_m)$, and let γ be a quantity of interest which is well-defined for every model s. The posterior distribution of γ is

$$p(\gamma \mid \mathbf{y}) = \sum_{s}^{m} p(\gamma \mid M_s, \mathbf{y}) p(M_s \mid \mathbf{y}),$$

where $p(\gamma \mid M_s, \mathbf{y})$ is the posterior of γ under the sth model and

$$p(M_s \mid \mathbf{y}) = \frac{f(\mathbf{y} \mid M_s)p(M_s)}{\sum_j f(\mathbf{y} \mid M_j)p(M_j)}.$$

This approach is referred to as Bayesian model averaging, which is not unlike the ensembling approaches described in Volume 2, Chapter 19, "A Causal Inference Framework" [129]. The basis for this approach, like ensemble methods, is that model averaging has better average predictive ability than using a single model. Some challenges related to this approach include the large number of models to consider, knowing what class of models to consider, determining how to select a prior distribution for each model, and the computational complexity.

25.4 Causal Inference Assumptions

Volume 2, Chapter 19, "A Causal Inference Framework," described the assumptions required when making causal statements. Some strategies for assessing some of the key assumptions were discussed. Here, we provide a summary of approaches.

25.4.1 Representative Sample

Understanding the sample used to make inferences fundamentally impacts conclusions. If the sample is thought of as randomly obtained from some larger population,[2] Comparing any information available between the larger population and the sample is a first step. In provider profiling, there are different sampling units, providers, and patients, and these both require consideration when making conclusions. Provider-level characteristics and patient-level characteristics for the sample are commonly summarized, but these are often not compared to the larger population of providers and patients. Construction of a CONSORT (Consolidated Standards of Reporting Trials) flow diagram that describes the number of experimental units (providers) potentially eligible for study inclusion, the number excluded due to any study constraints (e.g., not having the minimum number of patients), the number of remaining providers, and the number analyzed is helpful. Figure 25.3 presents the type of information typically included in a CONSORT diagram, modified for the profiling setting. While this information is used for *reporting* the flow of experimental units to the analytical sample, it points to several useful *comparisons*: A comparison of the analytical sample with the enrollment sample and with the allocated sample based on both provider and patient characteristics.

25.4.2 Positivity and Overlap

Standardized mean differences (SMD) can be used to assess the balance across providers for each confounder. This statistic is measured in standard deviations and thus can be used for any type of outcome metric. With two treatment groups, let $\bar{x}_{1p}$ and $\bar{x}_{2p}$ denote the mean of the pth covariate in the two groups, and let s^2_{ip} denote the within-group sample variance of the pth confounder in group i,

$$s^2_{ip} = \frac{1}{n_i - 1} \sum_{j=1}^{n_i} (x_{ipj} - \bar{x}_{ipj})^2,$$

where the summation is over patients indexed by j. The SMD is

$$\delta_p = \frac{\bar{x}_{1p} - \bar{x}_{2p}}{\sqrt{(s^2_{1p} + s^2_{2p})/2}}. \qquad (25.6)$$

The SMD does not *test* for differences in means between two groups; rather, it is a measure of differences between the two distributions as reflected by their locations. The larger δ_p, the more imbalance between the two groups based on

[2] It is not necessary to view the sample from a superpopulation. The potential outcomes from the population could be viewed as fixed, and only the treatment assignment is random. See Hinkelmann and Kempthorne [130].

confounder p. In general, SMDs < 0.20 are considered small [131]. Larger values suggest that the linear predictor in a glm will not be adequate to account for differences. Positivity and overlap are assessed for the causal parameter. The measures above are computed when interest centers in the average treatment effect. If interest is on the average treatment effect on those in group 1, then

$$\delta_p = \frac{\bar{x}_{1p} - \bar{x}_{2p}}{\sqrt{s_{1p}^2}}. \tag{25.7}$$

A comparison of the dispersion in the two groups uses the logarithm of the ratio of the two sample standard deviations,

$$\log(s_{1p}) - \log(s_{2p}), \tag{25.8}$$

where, again, larger values suggest differences in the distributions between the two groups. Differences in confounder distributions can be compared using the Kolmogorov–Smirnov statistic, κ, that compares the empirical distribution (ed) function between groups,

$$\mathrm{ed}(x_{1p}) = \frac{\sum_{j=1}^{N} I(Group_{ij} = 1) I(X_{1p} \leqslant x)}{\sum_{j=1}^{N} I(Group_{ij} = 1)} \text{ and } \kappa_p = \sup_x \mid \mathrm{ed}(x_{1p}) - \mathrm{ed}(x_{2p}) \mid, \tag{25.9}$$

where $I(Group_{ij} = 1)$ takes the value of 1 if the condition is true and 0 otherwise.

Figure 25.3 CONSORT flow diagram. I denotes the number of providers and n is the total number of patients.

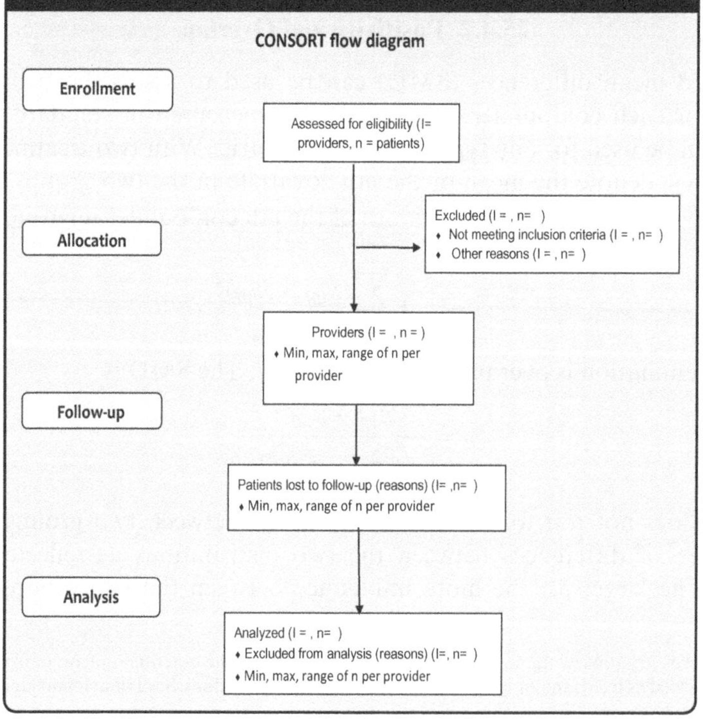

Figure 25.4 Overlap distributions for probability of treatment at Hospital 1

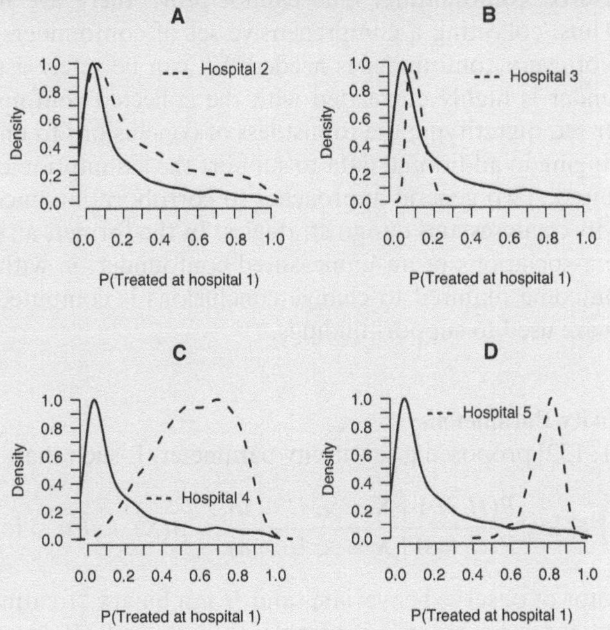

For provider profiling, interest is generally in the ATT, comparing the balance for those treated by provider i with those not treated by provider i. In this instance,

$$\delta_p = \frac{\bar{x}_{ip} - \bar{x}_{i*p}}{s_{ip}} \text{ and } \kappa_p = \sup_x \mid \text{ed}(x_{ip}) - \text{ed}(x_{i*p}) \mid, \; i \neq i*. \tag{25.10}$$

As the number of providers increases, summaries (mean, minimum, maximum) and graphical displays of κ_p and δ_p will be required.

Overlap refers to the balance between groups in the probability of assignment to each group and is assessed using the same metrics as above, but rather than examining balance in the confounder, balance in the logit of the estimated propensity score is examined. For provider profiling, recall $q_{ij} = p_{ij}(H_{ij} = 1 \mid \mathbf{x}_{ij})$ (see Volume 2, Chapter 19, "A Causal Inference Framework"), so the SMD and Kolmogorov–Smirnov statistic evaluate the balance of logit(q_{ij}). Values of these statistics can be used to understand case-mix differences across providers. Figure 19.1, from Volume 2, Chapter 19, (reproduced below as Figure 25.4) provided an illustration of pairwise overlap of five different hospitals with another hospital (Hospital 1). There appears to be good overlap between patients treated at Hospitals 1 and 2 (A), while there are large differences between Hospital 3 and Hospital 1 (B) and Hospital 5 and Hospital 1 (D). There is overlap between Hospital 4 and Hospital 1, although the two hospitals, on average, treat patients at different ends of the distributions.

25.4.3 Unconfoundedness

The most frequent concern when assessing cause and effect with observational data is unmeasured confounding. One cannot *prove* there are no unmeasured confounders. Thus, collecting a comprehensive set of confounders is a minimum requirement. Not every confounder is needed if it can be safely assumed that the missing confounder is highly correlated with the collected confounders. Given a rich confounder set, quantifying the robustness of conclusions to unmeasured confounding or bringing in additional data to support the assumption of unconfoundedness are required. Two general approaches to corroborating unconfoundedness include sensitivity analyses and design strategies. In the former, an estimate of the strength of the associations of an unmeasured confounder, u, with the treatment and with the outcome required to change conclusions is computed; in the latter, additional data are used to support findings.

25.4.3.1 Sensitivity Parameters

Rosenbaum [31, 132] proposed a sensitivity parameter, Γ such that

$$\log\left(\frac{1}{\Gamma}\right) \leqslant \log\frac{P(H=1 \mid \mathbf{X}=\mathbf{x}, U=u)}{P(H=0 \mid \mathbf{X}=\mathbf{x}, U=u)} = \beta(\mathbf{X}) + \beta_1 u \leqslant \log(\Gamma), \quad (25.11)$$

where $\mathbf{X}$ is a vector of observed covariates and H is a binary "treatment" indicator. When the treatment assignment is ignorable, then $\beta_1 = 0$. If $\beta_1 \neq 0$, then odds for two people with identical values of the observed covariates but different values of the unmeasured covariate differ by at most $\exp(\beta_1(u - u*))$. For example, if $\Gamma = 2$, then two subjects who appear similar on the same covariates could differ in their odds of receiving treatment by as much as a factor of 2. Rosenbaum developed bounds on the p-values associated with testing for a treatment effect [132]. The findings are insensitive to unmeasured confounding if (relatively) large values of Γ are required to change the p-value from "significant" to "non-significant." Of course, small treatment effects exist, and sensitivity to modest values of Γ does not mean that bias is present; rather, if it was present, the study conclusions would change. The authors demonstrated that assuming the scale of the unmeasured parameter is uniform between 0 and 1 in Eq. (25.11) sufficiently covers all other scales.

Vanderweele and Arah [133] proposed another parameter, denoted as an E-value (*Evidence for causality*). This parameter is the minimum strength of association on the risk ratio scale that an unmeasured confounder would need to have with both the treatment and the outcome to explain away a specific treatment–outcome association, conditional on the measured covariates. In this sense, it is close to ideas motivating Eq. (25.11) but makes no assumptions about the structure of the relationship between unmeasured confounders and the outcome or treatment. The approach assumes that the causal parameter is a risk ratio, ρ, and defines the E-value as

$$E = \rho + \sqrt{\rho \times (\rho - 1)}. \quad (25.12)$$

If the risk ratio is 2, then the E-value is $2 + \sqrt{2} = 3.4$, interpreted to mean that the risk ratio of 2 could be explained entirely by an unmeasured confounder (beyond all other confounders in the model) having a risk ratio of 3.4 with *both* the treatment and the outcome. Formulas for additional causal parameters, such as odds ratios, risk differences, and hazard ratios, are reported in VanderWeele and Ding [134].

25.4.3.2 Design Strategies

Other strategies used to support the unconfoundedness assumption adopted in assessing treatment effectiveness involve the use of falsification outcomes or the inclusion of multiple control groups. A falsification outcome (negative control outcome) should not differ across treatment arms. If differences are observed in the falsification outcomes among treatment arms, then unmeasured confounders are likely at play [135–137]. The problem is that finding such an outcome is often elusive in general. In studies where an outcome is measured at baseline, before any treatment, we would expect no differences among treatment arms. However, frequently, negative control outcomes are measured on a different scale than the primary outcome of interest. For instance, when assessing the occurrence of cardiometabolic morbidities associated with different antipsychotic drugs, flu vaccination rates could be used as negative control outcomes given that the choice of different antipsychotics should not impact the likelihood of flu vaccination. If a negative control outcome is identified, this information can also be used to correct the causal effect to unmeasured confounding [138].

Multiple control groups [139] may also be used to corroborate a finding. Suppose there are two control groups, and after adjusting for observed confounding, a difference in the average outcomes between the two control groups is observed. This implies that *at least one* of the control groups differs from the treated group based on an unmeasured confounder. Letting $H = 2$ and $H = 3$ denote two control groups, $H = 0$ denote the treated group, and U an unmeasured confounder, then either

$$\begin{aligned} &P(U \mid H = 0, \mathbf{X}) \neq P(U \mid H = 1, \mathbf{X}) \text{ or } P(U \mid H = 0, \mathbf{X}) \neq P(U \mid H = 2, \mathbf{X}) \\ &\text{if } P(Y \mid H = 1, \mathbf{X}) \neq P(Y \mid H = 2, \mathbf{X}). \end{aligned} \tag{25.13}$$

[140] demonstrate how to use the difference in outcomes between multiple control groups to correct the causal effect for unmeasured bias.

How does one select additional control groups? Try to find two groups that are likely to differ based on the unmeasured confounder U. For example, when profiling hospital CABG surgery programs, unmeasured case-mix is always a concern. Because teaching hospitals are thought to treat more complex cases than non-teaching hospitals, but in of themselves, should not affect outcomes, differences in 30-day surgical mortality between teaching and non-teaching hospitals may suggest unmeasured confounding. Stuart and Rubin [140] have exploited multiple control groups to adjust for unmeasured differences.

25.4.4 Stable Unit Treatment Value

This assumption is an *exclusion restriction* assumption required to identify a causal parameter and is justified on the basis of information external to the study. Two assumptions are involved: One asserts that multiple versions of the treatment are not permitted. In other words, the treatments are clearly defined, and everyone assigned a particular treatment received the same version of that treatment. For instance, is an antipsychotic drug taken orally the same as the injectable version? In a study comparing CABG surgery to percutaneous coronary intervention (PCI), is PCI delivered the same way for all patients? Some patients undergoing PCI may have a coronary stent implanted, while others may have a drug-eluting balloon utilized. CABG surgery may be performed more successfully by some surgeons but not by others. One solution to the multiple treatment version problem is to redefine the treatments [141]. For instance, surgery could be compared to PCI with coronary stents and PCI with drug-eluting balloons.

The other piece of SUTVA is the no interference assumption or the no spillover effect: The treatment I receive does not impact your outcome. If this assumption is violated, one could redefine the units. For instance, the no interference assumption is violated at the individual patient level but likely reasonable at, say, the hospital level when assessing provider quality [142].

25.5 Summary

Assessing the appropriateness of model fit in hierarchical generalized linear models is more complex than in the generalized linear model because of the multiple levels of the hierarchy, each of which may be linked to covariates. Thus, the functional form of the relationships between the covariates and "outcome" at each level of the hierarchy requires assessment, as do the distributional assumptions. A key point to keep in mind when profiling providers is that the goal is not to obtain a model that fits all the data well; rather, it is to determine how far units are from a standard using a reasonable model. Thus, if one provider is far from all other providers, permitting a longer-tailed distribution may mask real differences in provider performance.

Methods for inferring causal effects in the setting of multi-valued treatments require a clear statement on the causal parameter of interest, which may involve assessing if there are differences across providers had all patients been randomized to providers or assessing if a provider's outcomes are different from what was expected given the provider's case-mix. Determination of covariate balance and overlap differ, between these two scenarios. Approaches to assessing the sensitivity of results to unmeasured confounders were described; bounds in plausible ranges for causal effects can be determined, and the interested reader should see Manski [143].

CHAPTER TWENTY-SIX

Future Directions

Given the familiarity and wide availability of regression modeling, parametric modeling combined with direct or indirect standardization is the most common approach for profiling healthcare providers. In many settings, the statistical approaches described in previous chapters are appropriate. In other settings, parametric models may be misspecified if a large number of risk factors is needed to avoid unmeasured confounding. Approaches that relax parametric assumptions, briefly introduced in Chapter 19, are safer. In this final chapter, we describe a sample of approaches for inferring provider quality using semiparametric and nonparametric tools from the causal inference literature. These approaches differ in two distinct ways from the earlier chapters. First, they do not use direct or indirect standardization, opting for a causal inference framework. Second, they relax parametric assumptions.

26.1 Causal Inference via Optimization

Chapter 19 introduced a causal inference framework for provider assessments as well as newer nonparametric approaches. Here, we briefly illustrate a constrained optimization algorithm for creating a causal estimator of the average treatment effect on the treated (ATT) to estimate each provider's effect—we are no longer using regression modeling, so no longer focused on the conditional average treatment effect among the treated (CATT). Recalling the notation introduced earlier, where we let $H_j = i$ if patient j was treated in hospital i and 0 otherwise. The idea is to develop a set of weights subject to some balancing and complexity conditions.

Entropy balancing weights (Hainmueller [144]) are designed to achieve exact balance of covariate distributions between a treatment and comparison arm. In the quality setting, the treatment group is a specific hospital (the *target*), and the comparison group is formed by pooling patients from all other hospitals. The weights, w_j, for the comparison group, are obtained by solving the following optimization problem

$$\min_{w} \underbrace{\sum_{H_j \neq i} w_j \log\left(\frac{w_j}{q_j}\right)}_{\text{Kullback–Leibler}} \text{ such that } \underbrace{\sum_{H_j \neq i} w_j \psi_{r_j}(X_j) = (X_j - \mu_j)^r}_{\text{Imbalance}}, \tag{26.1}$$

Figure 26.1 Distribution of standardized mean differences for each target hospital from its comparison group, unadjusted and entropy-weighted. Weights obtained using the ebalance package in R.

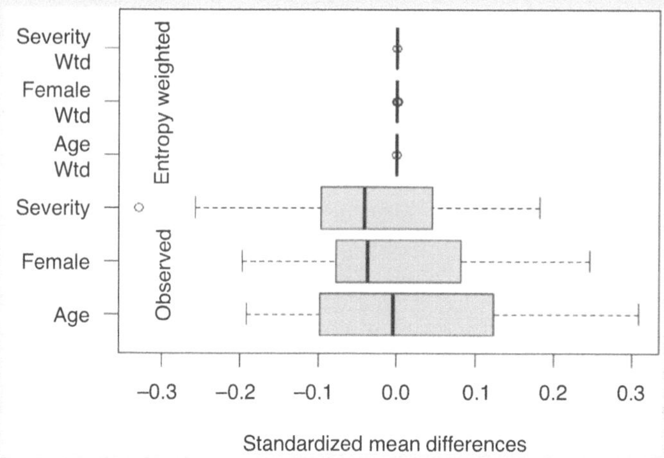

where $q_j = \frac{1}{\sum_{H_j \neq i} n_j}$, $q_j \geqslant 0$, are base weights, H_j denotes hospital, $\sum_{H_j \neq i} w_j = 1$, $w_j \geqslant 0$, and $r = 1, 2, \ldots, R$ denotes the number of constraints imposed on a covariate. The Kullback–Leibler measure represents the complexity measure of the weights to be minimized, basically minimizing the dispersion of the weights. Tan [145] showed that the entropy weights can be derived from a propensity-score model using a log-link. The imbalance constraints are user-specified. For instance, we could force the means, variances, or higher-order moments between the two groups to be equal. The positivity weight constraint ensures no extrapolation beyond the range of the observed covariates.

Returning to the patient satisfaction example (Chapter 21) for 1,977 patients treated at 20 hospitals presented earlier. The proportion responding satisfied across all hospitals was 0.11 and ranged 10-fold, from 0.034 to 0.33. Figure 26.1 displays the distribution of the standardized mean differences (SMD) of each target hospital from its respective comparison group for the three covariates considered in the example. The SMDs are shown for the observed means and the entropy-weighted means. The entropy-weighted means are effectively 0 because the algorithm exactly balances the means of the covariates. There are large differences before weighting, with SMDs of the observed covariates ranging from −0.3 to 0.3 across the 20 hospitals. In the example, given there are only three covariates, and we balanced only on the means; in real applications, the number of covariates is much larger, and constraints beyond the means are needed.

The provider-specific estimator (the ATT) is easily computed as

$$\frac{\frac{1}{n_i}\sum_{H_j=i} Y_j}{\sum_{H_j \neq i} \widehat{w}_j Y_j} = \left(\frac{O}{E}\right) \text{ or } \left(\frac{1}{n_i}\sum_{H_j=i} Y_j - \sum_{H_j \neq i} \widehat{w}_j Y_j\right).$$

Figure 26.2 Distribution of hospital-specific estimates for each target hospital from its comparison group using entropy-weighted ATT estimates. Weights obtained using the ebalance package in R.

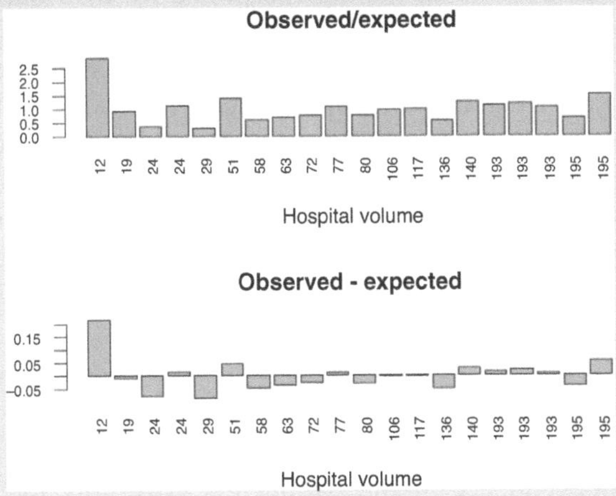

This process is then repeated for each hospital with patients reused in comparison groups for different targets (Figure 26.2).

26.1.1 Inference

For the difference between the observed and expected, define $\widehat{\mu}_{H_{j=i}} = \frac{1}{n_i}\sum_{j=1}^{n_i} Y_j$ for the target hospital and $\widehat{\mu}_{H_j \neq i} = \sum_{H_j \neq i} \widehat{w}_j Y_j$ for the comparison group. The variance of the difference in means, $\widehat{\tau}_{H_j=i} = \widehat{\mu}_{H_{j=i}} - \widehat{\mu}_{H_j \neq i}$, can be expressed as

$$\operatorname{Var}(\widehat{\tau}_{H_j=i}) = \operatorname{Var}(\widehat{\mu}_{H_j=i}) + \operatorname{Var}(\widehat{\mu}_{H_j \neq i})$$

by independence and can be decomposed into

$$\operatorname{Var}(\widehat{\tau}_{H_j=i}) = \frac{\sigma^2_{H_j=i}}{n_i} + \frac{\sigma^2_{H_j \neq i}}{n^{ess}_{H_j \neq i}}, \tag{26.2}$$

where $n^{ess}_{H_j \neq i} = \frac{1}{\sum_{H_j \neq i} w_j^2}$ represents the effective sample size (ESS) of the weighted comparison group. The ESS reflects the information content of the weighted sample, akin to an unweighted sample of the same size. Zhao and Percival [146] show that entropy balancing is doubly robust for linear outcome regression and logistic propensity score regression, and it reaches the asymptotic semiparametric variance bound when both regressions are correctly specified. Inference for the O/E can be conducted using the nonparametric bootstrap.

26.2 Bayesian Nonparametric Causal Inference Approaches

Bayesian semiparametric and nonparametric causal inference approaches combine machine learning with uncertainty quantification to permit the construction of causal parameter estimators. Recalling that the key issue in the causal inference setting is the missing counterfactual outcome, Rubin [147] argued Bayesian causal inference follows naturally from finding the predictive distribution of the counterfactual outcomes. Li et al. [148] provide an excellent review of Bayesian causal inference; for a review of nonparametric Bayesian causal inference, see Linero and Antonelli [149]. Oganisian and Roy [150] provide a practical guide to both parametric and nonparametric approaches; Spertus and Normand [151] provide an application to assessing the causal effect of drug eluting versus bare metal coronary stents.

In the Bayesian framework, combined with the standard causal inference assumptions, it is assumed that the joint distribution of the random variables, $\{H_j, Y_j(H_j), X_j\}$, conditional on the parameters $\tau = (\tau_H, \tau_Y, \tau_X)$, can be factored as

$$\underbrace{Pr(H_j \mid Y_j(H_j = i), Y_j(H_j \neq i), X_j; \tau_H)}_{\text{hospital assignment}} \underbrace{Pr(Y_j(H_j = i), Y_j(H_j \neq i) \mid X_j; \tau_Y)}_{\text{counterfactual outcomes}} \underbrace{Pr(X_j; \tau_X)}_{\text{confounders}}. \tag{26.3}$$

Assuming prior independence of the parameters governing the hospital assignment, counterfactual outcome, and confounder distribution, the posterior is proportional to

$$Pr(\tau_X) \prod_{j=1}^{N} Pr(X_j; \tau_X) Pr(\theta_H) \prod_{j=1}^{N} Pr(H_j \mid Y_j(H_j = i), Y_j(H_j \neq i), X_j; \tau_H)$$
$$\times\, Pr(\tau_Y) \prod_{j=1}^{N} Pr(Y_j(H_j = i), Y_j(H_j \neq i) \mid X_j; \tau_Y). \tag{26.4}$$

As in all Bayesian analyses, prior distributions are required for the components of τ. Li et al. [148] indicate that, depending on the causal parameter of interest, the hospital assignment model may not play a role in inference. We next discuss nonparametric Bayesian approaches and how the independence assumptions of the prior distributions in high-dimensional settings may cause problems.

26.2.1 The BART Approach

A Bayesian Additive Regression Trees (BART) is a Bayesian sum-of-trees model to approximate the mean of an outcome conditional on covariates introduced by Chipman et al. [152]. This is achieved by imposing a prior distribution that regularizes the fit by keeping the impact of each tree small. Without loss of generality, assume we have a binary outcome.[1] The BART model assumes that

$$P(Y_j = 1 \mid X_j) = \Phi\{G(X_j)\} : G(X_j) = \sum_{t=1}^{T} Tr(X_j, T_t, M_t), \tag{26.5}$$

[1] For continuous outcomes, assume additive errors, for example, $Y_j \mid X_j = \sum_{t=1}^{T} Tr(X_j, T_t, M_t) + \epsilon_t$.

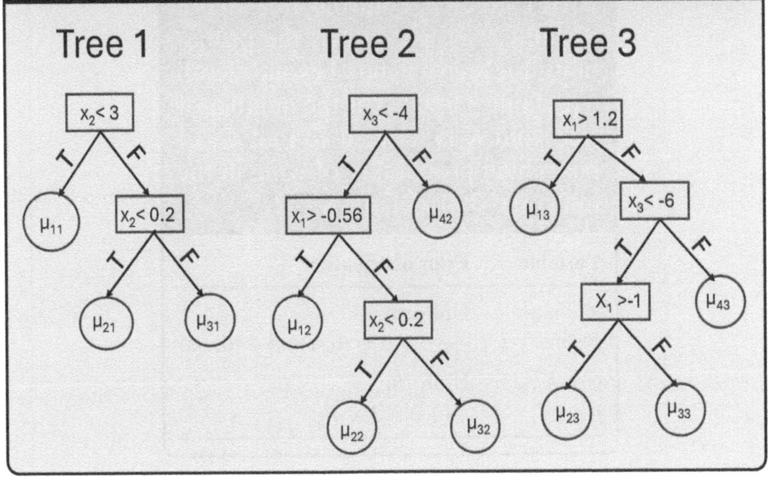

Figure 26.3 Example of three binary trees, part of BART.

where T_t is a binary decision tree, Φ denotes the probit link, and $M_t = (\mu_{1t}, \mu_{2t}, \ldots, \mu_{bt})$ is a vector of b expected outcomes in the terminal or leaf nodes. Figure 26.3 displays three trees that selected three variables, x_1, x_2, and x_3. Each tree, $Tr(X, T_t, M_t)$, is a collection of branch nodes, and each branch has a certain depth d that represents how far down the branch you travel to get to the leaf, M_t. In Figure 26.3, $M_3 = (\mu_{13}, \mu_{23}, \mu_{33}, \mu_{43})$. For each node on the branch, there is a threshold for a risk factor, X_j, denoted C, of the form $x_j \leqslant c$ or $x_j > c$. Tree 3, Figure 26.3, has depth 3, and splits first on x_1 using a threshold of $c = 1.2$, then x_3 using a threshold of $c = -6$, and finally on x_1 again using $c = -1$. The prior distributions for each tree are assumed independent and symmetric such that

$$P((T_1, M_1), (T_2, M_2), \ldots, (T_T, M_T)) = \prod_{t=1}^{T} p(T_t, M_t) = \prod_{t=1}^{T} p(M_t \mid T_t) p(T_t)$$

$$\text{with } p(M_t \mid T_t) = \prod_{k \in M_t} p(\mu_{kt} \mid T_t),$$

so for each tree, the prior is a product of the prior for the tree, $p(T_t)$, and the prior for the expected outcomes in the leaves given the tree, $p(T_t, M_t)$.

The prior for the tree involves iteratively selecting a variable, determining if a node will be a branch or a leaf, and if a branch, what splitting rule and threshold will be used. The number of trees is typically specified by the user, although this could be treated as a parameter to be estimated. BART's regularization encourages a small number of low-order interactions. Table 26.1 describes the regularization priors used in the BART R package.

BART models for other outcomes have been proposed, including Poisson, multionomial, negative binomial, and survival. BART is very flexible and requires no prior knowledge about how risk factors are parametrically related. The interested reader should consult Tan and Roy [153] who provide an excellent tutorial on BART.

Table 26.1 Prior distribution for BART tree. β controls tree depth (default = 2); γ controls the probability the tree extends beyond depth 0 (default = 0.95). T is the number of trees and K is selected so that $G(X)$ has a high probability of lying in the interval (–3,3); default K = 2.

Variable	Prior distribution
$X_j \mid d$	Uniform
$Branch \mid d$	$\frac{\gamma}{(1+d)^{\beta}}$, $\alpha \in (0,1)$, $\beta \in [0,\infty)$
$C_j \mid X_j, d$	Uniform
$\mu_{kt} \mid T_t$	$N(0, 3.0/K\sqrt{T})$

26.2.1.1 Inference

Inference is based on the posterior distribution of the parameters using simulation-based methods via a Markov Chain Monte Carlo back-fitting algorithm. Posterior means or medians can be calculated based on the draws, as can 100(1-α) posterior intervals. The Bayesian machinery easily permits posterior distributions of functions of parameters to be estimated with corresponding uncertainty quantification.

26.2.2 BART for Causal Inference

Hill [154] introduced the use of BART for causal inference. This was a particularly clever idea for several reasons. First, BART is flexible, providing a robust framework for inference. Nonlinear relationships between confounders and outcomes are easily incorporated without prespecification. Second, given its Bayesian framework, it naturally provides a principled approach to uncertainty quantification. Third, more confounders than a typical regression model can be handled.

Hill [154] proposed fitting a single BART model where one of the covariates is the treatment indicator, assuming ignorability of the treatment assignment,

$$E(Y_j(H_j = i) \mid X_j) = E(Y_j \mid H_j = i, X_j) = \Phi\{G(H_j = i, X_j)\}. \tag{26.6}$$

For the profiling setting, we select each hospital as the target treatment and pool all other patients into a comparison group to obtain

$$\widehat{\tau}_{H_j=i} = \frac{1}{n_i} \sum_{H_j=i} \left(\Phi^{-1}\{\widehat{G}(H_j = i, X_j)\} - \Phi^{-1}\{\widehat{G}(H_j \neq i, X_j)\} \right), \tag{26.7}$$

where the quantity in Eq. (26.7) may be a posterior mean or median or some other quantity estimated from the joint posterior. Credible intervals or the full posterior distribution for the estimate are easily calculated from draws using Markov Chain Monte Carlo simulation strategies.

A problem with all regression modeling, particularly modeling in high dimensions, is the lack of overlap, and this problem is exacerbated as the number of risk factors is increased. In the Bayesian nonparametric setting, Linero [155] demonstrated that when assuming the parameters governing the potential outcomes and treatment assignment mechanisms are independent (Eq. 26.4), many of the Bayesian regularization prior distributions, including that used in BART, are strongly informative. The solution is to include the propensity score in the regression model and this is next discussed.

26.2.3 Bayesian Causal Forest

In addition to the problem identified by Linero [155], Hahn et al. [156] also identified an additional problem with Bayesian regularization priors, which they characterized as *regularization induced confouding* (Box 26.1): The regularized prior used may cause bias in high dimensions for causal inference, which Linero recognized and inadequate control of variance of average treatment effects related to possible treatment effect heterogeneity.

Rather than fitting a single BART model, Hahn et al. [156] proposed fitting two BART models,

$$\begin{aligned} E(Y_j \mid H_j, X_j) &= \underbrace{E(Y_j \mid H_j \neq i, \widehat{\pi}(X_j))}_{\textit{prognostic}} + \underbrace{\left\{E(Y_j \mid H_j = i, X_j) - E(Y_j \mid H_j \neq i, X_j)\right\} H_j}_{\textit{provider effect}} \\ &= f_0(X_j, \widehat{\pi}(X_j)) + \underbrace{f_1(X_j)H_j}_{\textit{heterogeneity}}, \end{aligned} \tag{26.8}$$

where $\widehat{\pi}(X_j)$ is the estimated propensity score. Here, f_k is a sum-of-trees model, such as, $\Phi\{G(X)\}$. Separate BART prior distributions are given to f_0 and f_1. The inclusion of the propensity score in the model limits the regression model from erroneously, attributing the effect of confounders to the treatment variable. The first term, f_0, is a prognostic component that represents, in the profiling setting, the conditional mean outcome unrelated to the provider. The second term, f_1, is the (conditional) provider effect, which may vary by case-mix.

The prior distribution for f_0 is the same as that described in Table 26.1. For f_1, the authors suggest stronger regularization, setting $\beta = 3$ and $\gamma = 0.25$ (Table 26.1). For continuous outcomes, a half-Cauchy over the scale of the leaf parameters with prior median equal to twice the marginal standard deviation of Y_j for f_0 is used; a half-Normal prior for the scale of f_1 using the prior median to the marginal standard deviation of differences in the observed data are used.

Box 26.1 Regularization-induced confounding

A problem that occurs in Bayesian nonparametric high-dimensional methods when regularization to control the complexity of the nuisance parameters indirectly regularizes important causal parameters.

26.2.4 Other Nonparametric Prior Distributions

The Bayesian nonparametric approaches discussed thus far have assumed a semiparametric regression model of the form

$$Y_j = g_j(X_j) + \epsilon_j;\ \epsilon_j \sim N(0, \sigma^2), \tag{26.9}$$

where we used $\sigma^2 = 1$ for the (nonparametric) probit model and a BART prior distribution for $g_j(X_j)$. Other nonparametric prior distributions are available, including Gaussian processes, Dirichlet processes, and spike-and-slab priors for high-dimensional models. Gaussian processes generalize the multivariate normal distribution from vectors to functions. When $g_j(X)$ is a tree, the BART and Gaussian processes are the same when conditioning on the tree structures. Dirichlet processes are mixture models around a base distribution and are flexible. A spike-and-slab prior for g_j is a mixture of a point-mass distribution at 0 having a Bernoulli distribution with probability π_j (the spike) and $1 - \pi_j$ of a Gaussian process (the slab) and has been proposed for the high-dimensional setting.

26.3 Summary

Provider profiling has traditionally resided outside of the causal inference framework, relying on indirect standardization via parametric regression. The two emerging issues discussed in this chapter are viewing profiling from the causal lens and adopting Bayesian semiparametric and nonparametric approaches. We provided a single example of an optimization-based approach—other approaches were discussed in Chapter 19, and their many advantages were discussed there. The literature on optimization-based causal inference approaches is vast and beyond the scope of this book. The Bayesian approaches described in this chapter provide conditional estimates there is nothing to prevent the method from extrapolating over areas where there is no common support. The additional benefit of uncertainty quantification with the Bayesian nonparametric approaches and the ease of examining functions of parameters, however, should not be understated. Fully Bayesian nonparametric approaches to provider profiling, particularly incorporating sensitivity analyses, determining areas of common support, and developing methods to reliably estimate the sample average treatment effects (SATE), are worth pursuing.

Bibliography

[1] Shahian, D. M., Silverstein, T., Lovett, A. F., Wolf, R. E., and Normand, S. L. T. Comparison of clinical and administrative data sources for hospital coronary artery bypass graft surgery report cards. *Circulation*, 115:1518–1527, 2007.

[2] Goldstein, H. Multilevel covariance component models. *Biometrika*, 74:430–431, 1987.

[3] National Quality Forum. NQF measure testing, 2011. Accessed July 23, 2011 at www.qualityforum.org/Measuring_Performance/Submitting_Standards/Measure_Evaluation_Criteria.aspx.

[4] Drozda, J. P., Jr., Hagan, E. P., Mirro, M. J., Peterson, E. D., and Wright, J. S. ACCF 2008 health policy statement on principles for public reporting of physician performance data: A Report of the American College of Cardiology Foundation Writing Committee to develop principles for public reporting of physician performance data. *Journal of the American College of Cardiology*, 51:1993–2001, 2008.

[5] Krumholz, H. M., Brindis, R. G., Brush, J. E., et al. Standards for statistical models used for public reporting of health outcomes: An American Heart Association Scientific Statement from the Quality of Care and Outcomes Research Interdisciplinary Writing Group: Co-sponsored by the Council on Epidemiology and Prevention and the Stroke Council. Endorsed by the American College of Cardiology Foundation. *Circulation*, 113:456–462, 2006.

[6] Battelle. Partnership for Quality Measurement, 2025. https://p4qm.org/.

[7] Battelle. Partnership for Quality Measurement. Endorsement & Maintenance: What endorsement means, 2025. https://p4qm.org/EM.

[8] Battelle. Partnership for Quality Measurement: E&M Projects, 2025. https://p4qm.org/EM/projects.

[9] Battelle. Partnership for Quality Measurement. A beginners guide to the Battelle endorsement & maintenance process, 2025. https://p4qm.org/sites/default/files/material/EM-Beginners-Guide.pdf.

[10] Osswald, B. R., Tochtermann, U., Schweiger, P., et al. Minimal early mortality in CABG – Simply a question of surgical quality? *The Thoracic and Cardiovascular Surgeon*, 50:276–280, 2002.

[11] Osswald, B. R., Blackstone, E. H., Tochtermann, U., Thomas, G., Vahl, C. F., and Hagl, S. The meaning of early mortality after CABG. *European Journal of Cardio-Thoracic Surgery*, 15(4):401–407, 1999.

[12] Hannan, E. L., Kilburn, H., O'Donnell, J. F., Lukacik, G., and Shields, E. P. Adult open heart surgery in New York state: An analysis of risk factors and hospital

mortality rates. *The Journal of the American Medical Association*, 264(21):2768–2774, 1990.

[13] Green, J. and Wintfeld, N. Report cards on cardiac surgeons. Assessing New York state's approach. *The New England Journal of Medicine*, 332:1229–1232, 1995.

[14] Hannan, E. L., Sarrazin, M. S., Doran, D. R., and Rosenthal, G. E. Provider profiling and quality improvement efforts in coronary artery bypass graft surgery: The effect on short-term mortality among Medicare beneficiaries. *Medical Care*, 41:1164–1172, 2003.

[15] Silber, J. H., Rosenbaum, P. R., Schwartz, J. S., Ross, R. N., and Williams, S. V. Evaluation of the complication rate as a measure of quality of care in coronary artery bypass graft surgery. *The Journal of the American Medical Association*, 274(4):317–323, 1995.

[16] Normand, S. L. T., Wolf, R. E., Ayanian, J. Z., and McNeil, B. J. Assessing the accuracy of hospital clinical performance measures. *Medical Decision Making*, 27(1):9–20, 2007.

[17] Steyerberg, E. *Clinical Prediction Models: A Practical Approach to Development, Validation, and Updating, Second Edition*. Springer Nature Switzerland AG, Cham, 2019.

[18] Iezzoni, L. I. *Risk Adjustment for Measuring Health Care Outcomes*. Health Administration Press, Chicago, 4th ed., 2012.

[19] Holland, P. W. Statistics and causal inference. *Journal of the American Statistical Association*, 81:945–960, 1986.

[20] Holland, P. W. and Rubin, D. B. Causal inference in retrospective studies. *Evaluation Review*, 12:203–231, 1988.

[21] Rothman, K. J. and Greenland, S. Causation and causal inference in epidemiology. *American Journal of Public Health*, 95:S144–S150, 2005.

[22] Rubin, D. B. Causal inference using potential outcomes: Design, modeling, decisions. *Journal of the American Statistical Association*, 100:322–331, 2005.

[23] Rubin, D. B. Comment: Neyman (1923) and causal inference in experiments and observational studies. *Statistical Science*, 5:472–480, 1990.

[24] Pearl, J. *Causality: Models, Reasoning, and Inference*. Cambridge University Press, Cambridge; New York, 2000.

[25] Hill, A. B. The environment and disease: Association or causation? *Proceedings of the Royal Society of Medicine*, 58:295–300, 1965.

[26] Gelman, A. and Hill, J. *Data Analysis Using Regression and Multilevel/Hierarchical Models*. Cambridge University Press, Cambridge; New York, 2007.

[27] Gelman, A. *Applied Bayesian Modeling and Causal Inference from Incomplete Perspectives*. Wiley, Chichester, 2004.

[28] Hernan, M. A. and Robins, J. M. Estimating causal effects from epidemiological data. *Journal of Epidemiology and Community Health*, 60:578–586, 2006.

[29] Little, R. J. and Rubin, D. B. Causal effects in clinical and epidemiological studies via potential outcomes: Concepts and analytical approaches. *Annual Review of Public Health*, 21:121–145, 2000.

[30] Robins, J. M. and Greenland, S. The role of model selection in causal inference from nonexperimental data. *American Journal of Epidemiology*, 123:392–402, 1986.

[31] Rosenbaum, P. R. *Observational Studies*. Sprinter Series in Statistics. Springer, New York, 2002.

[32] Rosenbaum, P. R. and Rubin, D. B. The central role of the propensity score in observational studies for causal effects. *Biometrika*, 70:41–55, 1983.

[33] Rosenbaum, P. R. and Rubin, D. B. Estimating the effects caused by treatments—Comment. *Journal of the American Statistical Association*, 79:26–28, 1984.

[34] Rothman, K. J., Greenland, S., and Lash, T. *Modern Epidemiology*. Lippincott Williams & Wilkins, Philadelphia, 2008.

[35] Rubin, D. B. Estimating causal effects of treatments in randomized and nonrandomized studies. *Journal of Educational Psychology*, 66:688–701, 1974.

[36] Rubin, D. B. Statistics and causal inference—Which ifs have causal answers. *Journal of the American Statistical Association*, 81:961–962, 1986.

[37] Rubin, D. B. Direct and indirect causal effects via potential outcomes. *Scandinavian Journal of Statistics*, 31:161–170, 2004.

[38] Rubin, D. B. The design versus the analysis of observational studies for causal effects: Parallels with the design of randomized trials. *Statistics in Medicine*, 26:20–36, 2007.

[39] Imbens, G. W. and Rubin, D. B. *Causal Inference for Statistics, Social, and Biomedical Sciences: An Introduction*. Cambridge University Press, New York, 2015.

[40] Rigdon, J. and Hudgens, M. G. Randomization inference for treatment effects on a binary outcome. *Statistics in Medicine*, 34(6):924–935, 2015.

[41] Kern, H. L., Stuart, E. A., Hill, J., and Green, D. P. Assessing methods for generalizing experimental impact estimates to target populations. *Journal of Research on Educational Effectiveness*, 9(1):103–127, 2016.

[42] Nguyen, T. Q., Ebnesajjad, C., Cole, S. R., and Stuart, E. A. Sensitivity analysis for an unobserved moderator in RCT-to-target-population generalization of treatment effects. *The Annals of Applied Statistics*, 11(1):225–247, 2017.

[43] Stuart, E. A., Cole, S. R., Bradshaw, C. P., and Leaf, P. J. The use of propensity scores to assess the generalizability of results from randomized trials. *Journal of the Royal Statistical Society: Series A (Statistics in Society)*, 174(2):369–386, 2011.

[44] Dababnah, S. and Parish, S. L. A comprehensive literature review of randomized controlled trials for parents of young children with autism spectrum disorder. *Journal of Evidence-Based Social Work*, 13(3):277–292, 2016.

[45] Hartman, E., Grieve, R., Ramsahai, R., and Sekhon, J. S. From sample average treatment effect to population average treatment effect on the treated: Combining experimental with observational studies to estimate population treatment effects. *Journal of the Royal Statistical Society. Series A (Statistics in Society)*, 178(3):757–778, 2015.

[46] Bareinboim, E. and Pearl, J. Transportability of causal effects: Completeness results. In *Proceedings of the Twenty-Sixth AAAI Conference on Artificial Intelligence*, pages 698–704. AAAI Press, 2012.

[47] Fleiss, J. L., Levin, B., and Paik, M. C. *Statistical Methods for Rates and Proportions*. John Wiley and Sons, New York, 3rd ed., 2003.

[48] Horvitz, D. G. and Thompson, D. J. A generalization of sampling without replacement from a finite universe. *Journal of the American Statistical Association*, 47(260):663–685, 1952.

[49] Li, F., Thomas, L. E., and Li, F. Addressing extreme propensity scores via the overlap weights. *American Journal of Epidemiology*, 188(1):250–257, 2019.

[50] Stuart, E. A. Matching methods for causal inference: A review and a look forward. *Statistical Science*, 25(1):1–21, 2010.

[51] Rosenbaum, P. R. and Silber, J. H. Matching and thick description in an observational study of mortality after surgery. *Biostatistics*, 2(2):217–232, 2001.

[52] Wang, Y. X. and Zubizarreta, J. R. Minimal dispersion approximately balancing weights: Asymptotic properties and practical considerations. *Biometrika*, 107(1):93–105, 2019.

[53] Ben-Michael, E., Feller, A., Hirshberg, D. A., and Zubizarreta, J. R. The balancing act in causal inference. *preprint*, page arXiv:2110.14831, 2021. https://api.semanticscholar.org/CorpusID:240070375.

[54] Chattopadhyay, A., Hase, C. H., and Zubizarreta, J. R. Balancing vs modeling approaches to weighting in practice. *Statistics in Medicine*, 39(24):3227–3254, 2020.

[55] Keele, L. J., Ben-Michael, E., Feller, A., Kelz, R., and Miratrix, L. Hospital quality risk standardization via approximate balancing weights. *The Annals of Applied Statistics*, 17(2):901–928, 2023.
[56] Han, L., Li, Y., Niknam, B. A., and Zubizarreta, J. R. Privacy-preserving, communication-efficient, and target-flexible hospital quality measurement. *Annals of Applied Statistics*, 18(2):1337–1359, 2024.
[57] Silber, J. H., Rosenbaum, P. R., Ross, R. N., Ludwig, J. M., Wang, W., Niknam, B. A., Mukherjee, N., Saynisch, P. A., Even-Shoshan, O., Kelz, R. R., and Fleisher, L. A. Template matching for auditing hospital cost and quality. *Health Services Research*, 49(5):1446–1474, 2014.
[58] Silber, J. H., Rosenbaum, P. R., Ross, R. N., Ludwig, J. M., Wang, W., Niknam, B. A., Saynisch, P. A., Even-Shoshan, O., Kelz, R. R., and Fleisher, L. A. A hospital-specific template for benchmarking its cost and quality. *Health Services Research*, 49(5):1475–1497, 2014.
[59] Silber, J. H., Rosenbaum, P. R., Ross, R. N., Ludwig, J. M., Wang, W., Niknam, B. A., Hill, A. S., Even-Shoshan, O., Kelz, R. R., and Fleisher, L. A. Indirect standardization matching: Assessing specific advantage and risk synergy. *Health Services Research*, 51(6):2330–2357, 2016.
[60] van der Laan, M. J., Polley, E. C., and Hubbard, A. E. Super learner. *Statistical Applications in Genetics and Molecular Biology*, 6:Article25, 2007.
[61] Spertus, J. V., Normand, S.-L. T., Wolf, R., Cioffi, M., Lovett, A., and Rose, S. Assessing hospital performance after percutaneous coronary intervention using big data. *Circulation: Cardiovascular Quality and Outcomes*, 9(6):659–669, 2016.
[62] Paddock, S. M. and Louis, T. A. Percentile-based empirical distribution function estimates for performance evaluation of healthcare providers. *Journal of the Royal Statistical Society, Series C (Applied Statistics)*, 60(4):575–589, 2011.
[63] Hausman, J. A. Specification tests in econometrics. *Econometrica*, 46(6):1251–1271, 1978.
[64] Pan, W. A note on the use of marginal likelihood and conditional likelihood in analyzing clustered data. *The American Statistician*, 56(3):171–174, 2002.
[65] Berlin, J. A., Kimmel, S. E., Ten Have, T. R., and Sammel, M. D. An empirical comparison of several clustered data approaches under confounding due to cluster effects in the analysis of complications of coronary angioplasty. *Biometrics*, 55(2):470–476, 1999.
[66] Neuhaus, J. and Kalbfleisch, J. Between and within-cluster covariate effects in the analysis of clustered data. *Biometrics*, 54:638–645, 1998.
[67] Ten Have, T. R., Landis, J. R., and Weaver, S. Association models for periodontal disease progression: A comparison of methods for clustered binary data. *Statistics in Medicine*, 14:413–429, 1995.
[68] Neuhaus, J., Kalbfleisch, J., and Hauck, W. Conditions for consistent estimation in mixed-effects models for binary matched pairs data. *Canadian Journal of Statistics*, 22:139–148, 1994.
[69] Kalbfleisch, J. D. and Wolfe, R. A. On monitoring outcomes of medical providers. *Statistics in Biosciences*, 5(2):286–302, 2013.
[70] Adams, J. L. *The Reliability of Provider Profiling: A Tutorial*. RAND Corporation, Santa Monica, CA, 2009. www.rand.org/pubs/technical_reports/TR653.html.
[71] He, K., Dahlerus, C., Xia, L., Li, Y., and Kalbfleisch, J. D. The profile inter-unit reliability. *Biometrics*, 76(2):654–663, 2020.
[72] Spiegelhalter, D. J., Abrams, K. R., and Myles, J. P. *Bayesian Approaches to Clinical Trials and Health-Care Evaluation*. Statistics in Practice. John Wiley & Sons, Chichester, 2004.

[73] Maritz, J. S. *Empirical Bayes Methods.* Monographs on Statistics and Applied Probability (Series) 35. Chapman and Hall, London; New York, 2nd ed., 1989.

[74] Laird, N. M. and Ware, J. H. Random-effects models for longitudinal data. *Biometrics*, 38(4):963–974, 1982.

[75] Morris, C. N. and Normand, S. L. Hierarchical models for combining information and for meta-analysis with discussion. In Bernardo, J. M., Berger, J. O., Dawid, A. P., and Smith, A. F. M., editors, *Bayesian Statistics 4: Proceedings of the Fourth Valencia International Meeting, April 15–20, 1991*, pages 321–344. Clarendon Press; Oxford University Press, Oxford, New York, 1992.

[76] Normand, S. L. T. Meta-analysis: Formulating, evaluating, combining, and reporting. *Statistics in Medicine*, 18(3):321–359, 1999.

[77] DuMouchel, W. and Normand, S. L. Computer modeling and graphical strategies for meta-analysis. In Berry, D. and Stangl, D., editors, *Meta-Analysis in Medicine and Health Policy*, pages 127–178. Taylor & Francis Group, New York, 2000.

[78] Dumouchel, W. H. and Harris, J. E. Bayes methods for combining the results of cancer studies in humans and other species. *Journal of the American Statistical Association*, 78(382):293–308, 1983.

[79] Lee, Y. and Nelder, J. A. Hierarchical generalized linear models. *Journal of the Royal Statistical Society: Series B (Methodological)*, 58(4):619–656, 1996.

[80] Daniels, M. J. and Gatsonis, C. Hierarchical generalized linear models in the analysis of variations in health care utilization. *Journal of the American Statistical Association*, 94(445):29–42, 1999.

[81] McCullagh, P. P. *Generalized Linear Models.* Monographs on Statistics and Applied Probability (Series). Chapman and Hall, London; New York, 1983.

[82] Carlin, B. P. and Louis, T. A. *Bayes and Empirical Bayes Methods for Data Analysis.* Chapman & Hall/CRC Texts in Statistical Science Series. Chapman & Hall/CRC, Boca Raton, 2nd ed., 2000.

[83] Lee, Y. J., Nelder, J. A., and Pawitan, Y. *Generalized Linear Models with Random Effects: Unified Analysis via H-likelihood.* Chapman & Hall/CRC Monographs on Statistics and Applied Probability. Chapman and Hall/CRC, Boca Raton, 2017.

[84] Jin, S. and Lee, Y. A review of h-likelihood and hierarchical generalized linear model. *WIREs Computational Statistics*, 13(5):e1527, 2021.

[85] Baker, F. B. *Item Response Theory: Parameter Estimation Techniques.* Statistics: A Series of Textbooks and Monographs. M. Dekker, New York, 1992.

[86] He, Y., Wolf, R. E., and Normand, S. T. Assessing geographical variations in hospital processes of care using multilevel item response models. *Health Services and Outcomes Research Methodology*, 10(3–4):111–133, 2010.

[87] Chen, W. H. and Thissen, D. Local dependence indexes for item pairs using item response theory. *Journal of Educational and Behavioral Statistics*, 22(3):265–289, 1997.

[88] Yen, W. M. Effects of local item dependence on the fit and equating performance of the three-parameter logistic model. *Applied Psychological Measurement*, 8(2):125–145, 1984.

[89] Sammel, M. D., Ryan, L. M., and Legler, J. M. Latent variable models for mixed discrete and continuous outcomes. *Journal of the Royal Statistical Society: Series B (Statistical Methodology)*, 59(3):667–678, 1997.

[90] Landrum, M. B., Normand, S. L. T., and Rosenheck, R. A. Selection of related multivariate means: Monitoring psychiatric care in the Department of Veterans Affairs. *Journal of the American Statistical Association*, 98:7–16, 2003.

[91] Cox, D. R. and Wermuth, N. Response models for mixed binary and quantitative variables. *Biometrika*, 79(3):441–461, 1992.

[92] Fitzmaurice, G. M. and Laird, N. M. Regression models for a bivariate discrete and continuous outcome with clustering. *Journal of the American Statistical Association*, 90(431):845–852, 1995.

[93] Catalano, P. J. and Ryan, L. M. Bivariate latent variable models for clustered discrete and continuous outcomes. *Journal of the American Statistical Association*, 87(419):651–658, 1992.

[94] Arminger, G. and Küsters, U. *Latent Trait Models with Indicators of Mixed Measurement Level*, pages 51–73. Springer US, Boston, MA, 1988.

[95] Dunson, D. B. Bayesian latent variable models for clustered mixed outcomes. *Journal of the Royal Statistical Society. Series B (Statistical Methodology)*, 62(2):355–366, 2000.

[96] Prentice, R. L. and Zhao, L. P. Estimating equations for parameters in means and covariances of multivariate discrete and continuous responses. *Biometrics*, 47(3):825–839, 1991.

[97] Zhao, L. P., Prentice, R. L., and Self, S. G. Multivariate mean parameter estimation by using a partly exponential model. *Journal of the Royal Statistical Society. Series B (Methodological)*, 54(3):805–811, 1992.

[98] Normand, S. L. T., Wolf, R. E., and McNeil, B. J. Discriminating hospital quality of care in the US. *Medical Decision Making*, 28:308–322, 2007.

[99] Landrum, M. B., Bronskill, S. E., and Normand, S. L. T. Analytic methods for constructing cross-sectional profiles of health care providers. *Health Services and Outcomes Research Methodology*, 1(1):23–48, 2000.

[100] Teixeira-Pinto, A. and Normand, S. L. Statistical methodology for classifying units on the basis of multiple-related measures. *Statistics in Medicine*, 27(9):1329–1350, 2008.

[101] Daniels, M. J. and Normand, S. L. Longitudinal profiling of health care units based on continuous and discrete patient outcomes. *Biostatistics*, 7(1):1–15, 2006.

[102] Tierney, L. and Kadane, J. Accurate approximations for posterior moments and marginal densities. *Journal of the American Statistical Association*, 81(393):82–86, 1986.

[103] Naylor, J. C. and Smith, A. F. M. Applications of a method for the efficient computation of posterior distributions. *Applied Statistics*, 31(3):214–225, 1982.

[104] Geweke, J. Bayesian inference in econometric models using Monte Carlo integration. *Econometrica*, 57(6):1317–1339, 1989.

[105] Devroye, L. *Non-uniform Random Variate Generation*. Springer-Verlag, New York, 1986.

[106] Besag, J. Spatial interaction and the statistical analysis of lattice systems. *Journal of the Royal Statistical Society. Series B, Methodological*, 36(2):192–236, 1974.

[107] Casella, G. and George, E. I. Explaining the Gibbs sampler. *The American Statistician*, 46(3):167–174, 1992.

[108] Geman, S. and Geman, D. Stochastic relaxation, Gibbs distributions, and the Bayesian restoration of images. *IEEE Transactions on Pattern Analysis and Machine Intelligence*, PAMI-6(6):721–741, 1984.

[109] Schervish, M. J. and Carlin, B. P. On the convergence of successive substitution sampling. *Journal of Computational and Graphical Statistics*, 1(2):111–127, 1992.

[110] Gelfand, A. E. and Smith, A. F. M. Sampling-based approaches to calculating marginal densities. *Journal of the American Statistical Association*, 85(410):398–409, 1990.

[111] Metropolis, N., Rosenbluth, A. W., Rosenbluth, M. N., Teller, A. H., and Teller, E. Equation of state calculations by fast computing machines. *The Journal of Chemical Physics*, 21(6):1087–1092, 1953.

[112] Hastings, W. K. Monte Carlo sampling methods using Markov chains and their applications. *Biometrika*, 57(1):97–109, 04 1970.

[113] Chib, S. and Greenberg, E. Understanding the Metropolis-Hastings algorithm. *The American Statistician*, 49(4):327–335, 1995.

[114] Gelfand, A. E., Sahu, S. K., and Carlin, B. P. Efficient parametrisations for normal linear mixed models. *Biometrika*, 82(3):479–488, 1995.

[115] Gelman, A. and Rubin, D. B. Inference from iterative simulation using multiple sequences. *Statistical Science*, 7(4):457–472, 1992.

[116] Geyer, C. J. Practical Markov Chain Monte Carlo. *Statistical Science*, 7(4):473–483, 1992.

[117] Raftery, A. E. and Lewis, S. How many iterations in the Gibbs sampler? In Bernardo, J. M., Berger, J. O., Dawid, A. P., and Smith, A. F. M., editors, *Bayesian Statistics 4: Proceedings of the Fourth Valencia International Meeting, April 15–20, 1991*, pages 763–773. Clarendon Press; Oxford University Press, Oxford, New York, 1992.

[118] Cowles, M. K. and Carlin, B. P. Markov chain Monte Carlo convergence diagnostics: A comparative review. *Journal of the American Statistical Association*, 91(434):883–904, 1996.

[119] Nakajima, S., Watanabe, K., and Sugiyama, M. *Variational Bayesian Learning Theory*. Cambridge University Press, Cambridge, 2019.

[120] Geweke, J. Monte Carlo simulation and numerical integration. *Handbook of Computational Economics*, 1:731–800, 1995.

[121] Wedderburn, R. W. M. Quasi-likelihood functions, generalized linear models, and the Gauss-Newton method. *Biometrika*, 61(3):439–447, 1974.

[122] Morris, C. N. Parametric empirical Bayes inference: Theory and applications. *Journal of the American Statistical Association*, 78(381):47–55, 1983.

[123] Corbeil, R. R. and Searle, S. R. Restricted maximum likelihood (REML) estimation of variance components in the mixed model. *Technometrics*, 18(1):31–38, 1976.

[124] Bjørnstad, J. F. On the generalization of the likelihood function and the likelihood principle. *Journal of the American Statistical Association*, 91(434):791–806, 1996.

[125] Rue, H., Martino, S., and Chopin, N. Approximate Bayesian inference for latent Gaussian models by using integrated nested Laplace approximations. *Journal of the Royal Statistical Society: Series B (Statistical Methodology)*, 71(2):319–392, 2009.

[126] Jeffreys, H. *Theory of Probability*. Oxford University Press, Oxford, 3rd ed., 1961.

[127] Kass, R. E. and Raftery, A. E. Bayes factors. *Journal of the American Statistical Association*, 90(430):773–795, 1995.

[128] Schervish, M. J. *Theory of Statistics*. Springer Series in Statistics. Springer New York, New York, 1st ed., 1995.

[129] Hoeting, J. A., Madigan, D., Raftery, A. E., and Volinsky, C. T. Bayesian model averaging: A tutorial (with comments by M. Clyde, David Draper and E. I. George, and a rejoinder by the authors). *Statistical Science*, 14(4):382–417, 1999.

[130] Hinkelmann, K. and Kempthorne, O. *Design and Analysis of Experiments*. Wiley Series in Probability and Statistics. Wiley-Interscience, Hoboken, NJ, 2nd ed. 2008.

[131] McCaffrey, D. F., Griffin, B. A., Almirall, D., Slaughter, M. E., Ramchand, R., and Burgette, L. F. A tutorial on propensity score estimation for multiple treatments using generalized boosted models. *Statistics in Medicine*, 32(19):3388–3414, 2013.

[132] Rosenbaum, P. R. Sensitivity analysis for certain permutation inferences in matched observational studies. *Biometrika*, 74(1):13–26, 1987.

[133] Vanderweele, T. J. and Arah, O. A. Bias formulas for sensitivity analysis of unmeasured confounding for general outcomes, treatments, and confounders. *Epidemiology (Cambridge, Mass.)*, 22(1):42–52, 2011.

[134] VanderWeele, T. J. and Ding, P. Sensitivity analysis in observational research: Introducing the E-value. *Annals of Internal Medicine*, 167(4):268–274, 2017.

[135] Rosenbaum, P. R. The role of known effects in observational studies. *Biometrics*, 45(2):557–569, 1989.

[136] Lipsitch, M., Tchetgen Tchetgen, E., and Cohen, T. Negative controls: A tool for detecting confounding and bias in observational studies. *Epidemiology*, 21(3):383–388, 2010.

[137] Flanders, W. D., Klein, M., Darrow, L. A., Strickland, M. J., Sarnat, S. E., Sarnat, J. A., Waller, L. A., Winquist, A., and Tolbert, P. E. A method for detection of residual confounding in time-series and other observational studies. *Epidemiology*, 22(1):59–67, 2011.

[138] Tchetgen Tchetgen, E. The control outcome calibration approach for causal inference with unobserved confounding. *American Journal of Epidemiology*, 179(5):633–640, 2014.

[139] Rosenbaum, P. R. The role of a second control group in an observational study (with discussion). *Statistical Science*, 2(3):292–316, 1987.

[140] Stuart, E. A. and Rubin, D. B. Matching with multiple control groups with adjustment for group differences. *Journal of Educational and Behavioral Statistics*, 33(3):279–306, 2008.

[141] Cole, S. R. and Frangakis, C. E. The consistency statement in causal inference: A definition or an assumption? *Epidemiology*, 20(1):3–5, 2009.

[142] Tchetgen Tchetgen, E. J. and VanderWeele, T. J. On causal inference in the presence of interference. *Statistical Methods in Medical Research*, 21(1):55–75, 2012.

[143] Manski, C. F. Nonparametric bounds on treatment effects. *The American Economic Review*, 80(2):319–323, 1990.

[144] Hainmueller, J. Entropy balancing for causal effects: A multivariate reweighting method to produce balanced samples in observational studies. *Political Analysis*, 20(1):25–46, 2012.

[145] Tan, Z. Regularized calibrated estimation of propensity scores with model misspecification and high-dimensional data. *Biometrika*, 107(1):137–158, 2020.

[146] Zhao, Q. and Percival, D. Entropy balancing is doubly robust. *Journal of Causal Inference*, 5(1):1–19, 2017.

[147] Rubin, D. B. Bayesian inference for causal effects: The role of randomization. *The Annals of Statistics*, 6(1):34–58, 1978.

[148] Li, F., Ding, P., and Mealli, F. Bayesian causal inference: A critical review. *Philosophical Transactions of the Royal Society A*, 381(2247):20220153, 2023.

[149] Linero, A. R. and Antonelli, J. L. The how and why of Bayesian nonparametric causal inference. *Wiley Interdisciplinary Reviews: Computational Statistics*, 15:e1583, 2023.

[150] Oganisian, A. and Roy, J. A practical introduction to Bayesian estimation of causal effects: Parametric and nonparametric approaches. *Statistics in Medicine*, 40(2):518–551, 2021.

[151] Spertus, J. and Normand, S. Bayesian propensity scores for high-dimensional causal inference: A comparison of drug-eluting to bare-metal coronary stents. *Biometrical Journal*, 60(4):721–733, 2018.

[152] Chipman, H., George, E., and McCulloch, R. Bayesian additive regression trees. *The Annals of Applied Statistics*, 4(1):266–298, 2010.

[153] Tan, Y. V. and Roy, J. Bayesian additive regression tree and general BART model. *Statistics in Medicine*, 38(25):5048–5069, 2019.

[154] Hill, J. L. Bayesian nonparametric modeling for causal inference. *Journal of Computational and Graphical Statistics*, 20(1):217–240, 2011.

[155] Linero, A. R. In nonparametric and high-dimensional models, Bayesian ignorability is an informative priorbayesian regression trees for high-dimensional prediction and variable selection. *arXiv preprint*, arXiv:2111.05137, 2021.

[156] Hahn, P. R., Murray, M. S., and Carvalho, S. M. Bayesian regression tree models for causal inferences: Regularization, confounding, and heterogeneous effects (with discussion). *Bayesian Analysis*, 15(3):965–1056, 2020.

Index

Printed in the United Kingdom by TJ Clays Ltd.